HOLIST

FROM THE

PAN - AFRIKAN PERSPECTIVE

By

Iya Raet

Published by

UBUS Communications Systems

26070 Barhams Hill Road - Drewryville, VA 23844

publish@khabooks.com (704) 277-1462

FIRST EDITION - FIRST PRINTING

MAY, 2007

Edited by Rasheedah Parks, April Bogan, and Angelica Lindsay

Cover art: Maternity Dance © 2001 by Joshua Humphries

Published by Afrikan Holistic Living

ISBN# 1-56411- 500-3......YBBG# 0490

iyaraet@yahoo.com

www.afrikanparenting.com

printed in the U.S.A.
by
The Lumumba Book Printers
P. O. Box 9
Drewryville, VA 23844
(704) 277-1462 printing@khabooks.com

Disclaimer

This author is not a healthcare practitioner. Medical and health related concerns should be discussed with a physician. This book is not a substitution for medical advice.

Dedication

I dedicate this book to my son, Sun-Ra, you inspired and created this book. We lived this book together. Tua (thank you) for making this journey an easy one. Tua for being patient with your Iya. You are my creator. You offered me the chance to be reborn, allowing me to be the Mother Creatress, I was destined to be. You were once the hidden aspect of Ra, Amen, in my subconscious. Now, you shine your light so bright for the world to see. Tua for allowing me to bask in your rays.

Khonsu, the second baby born in my home, you taught me a very important lesson. We have to be prepared and vigilant in the pursuit of taking care of our babies. Tua for being so brave and strong.

I also dedicate this book to the children of hurricane Katrina.

Tua Neteru!
Ashe!

Table of Contents

Introduction 8

1 - The Womb 11

Vegan Diet during Pregnancy 16
Meditation 19
Preparation 21

2 - Know Your Options & Your Rights 25

Choosing an Obstetrician and Gynecologist, Midwife, or Unassisted Birth 25
Home, Birth center, or Hospital 28

3 - OB/GYNs and the Medicalization of Childbirth ...37

Prenatal Testing 37
Ultrasounds 39
Chemical Inductions 40
Narcotics 41
Epidurals 41
Electronic Fetal Monitoring (EFM) 42
Episiotomy 42
Caesarean 43
Physical and Psychological Affects of an over medicalized birth 44
Birth essays and poems from Iyas and Babas (Mothers and Fathers) 46

4 - Postpartum 58

The Placenta 58
Time of Rest 59
Circumcision 60
Baby Food 66
Cloth Diapering 69
Baby Wearing 75
Baby-sitting and Daycare 84

5 - Keeping Your Children Healthy 87

Vaccinations 87

Are Allopathic doctors right for you and your family? 94

Afrikan Medicinal Herbalism 96

Mother and Father are the child's primary care givers 105

Preparing For Emergencies 108

First Aid 110

Nutrition 111

6 - Toxic Free Home & Sustainable Living 122

Home Environment 122

Diodes 124

Natural Home Cleaning and Pest Control 124

Natural Personal Care 126

Toys for Children 127

The Toxic Black Hair Care Industry Poisoning Children and the Home 128

Television and Music 133

Family Rituals 134

Building Healthy Communities 136

Alternative Energy for Afrikans 137

7 - Education 142

Infant and Toddler Development 142

Afrikan–Centered Independent Schools and Homeschooling 144

Rites of Passage 152

Conclusion 156

Bibliography 160

Index 166

Acknowledgements

All praises and adoration to the ancestors, Neteru, Orishas, Abosom, and Loa!

I would like to thank my mother, Brenda, for allowing me to be her divine reflection.

Grandmom Dorothy and Aunt Linda, thanks for being there for me and Sun-Ra.

Felicia, thanks for being such a supportive God mother.

April, thanks for editing this book and being my best friend since the 4th grade. It all started with the big pack of crayola crayons with the sharpener, which we shared. Friends for 19 years!

Thanks to Angelica also for providing editing. You were the first to read my words, thanks for the support.

Jacqui, thanks for listening to me, providing fantastic readings, and encouragement.

Joshua, thanks for being a beautiful spirit and providing the beautiful art work for the book cover. Jah Bless!

Sis Basiymah, thank you for being such a great mentor.

Keidi Obi Awadu, thanks for providing daily education for me.

The urban shaman, Bro. Levi Hoodari SunguRa, thanks for sharing with me. You are truly a blessing to the Afrikan community.

Salithia, thanks for allowing me to take part in your beautiful homebirth. We have memories that will last a lifetime.

Tekeytha, thanks for being a good friend to Salithia and I. Thanks for revealing the spirit of Oya when it is time to make swift moves! We have to protect our babies!

Thank you Nana Okomfo Korantemaa Ayeboafo for providing the way for me to communicate with the ancestors that guided me during writing this book. This book was therapeutic and opened new doors. Just as the Abosom stated, there were long nights and a child wanting my constant attention, but I finished!

Kathy Hindle and Cristine Jude-Cox , my midwives, and my birth assistant Sheila, thanks for making my homebirth a beautiful experience!

Many blessings to the families who contributed:

Kameela Abdul Muhammad
Venus Paloma Rodriguez-McGregor
Roz Fattaleh
Dera and Emmanuel, Wanlov!
Aremisa Haile
Baiyina
Melinda Blythe
Rene
Sarpoma Sefa-Boakye
Yejide
Sha'Kmt
Salithia/Mut Rennenet
Desi and Mwenya Washington
Cris Nicole
Sa Mut Herr
Sherose
Akilah Muhammad
Cherie King

A beautiful friend of mine inspired me to write this book. He told me that everyone has at least one book in them, so here it is!

7

Introduction

This book is written from a Pan-Afrikanist perspective. Pan Afrikanism is the idea that all people of Afrikan descent regardless of whether they reside in the United States, United Kingdom, Puerto Rico, or Ghana, are focused on the advancement and liberation of all Afrikan people. Explored here is parenting for liberation of the Afrikan family.

There is a saying, "If you heal a woman, you heal a nation". I offer this book as a token of peace and healing. As a group of people, Afrikans hold much sickness, hurt, toxicity, and disease. These ailments are brought on by emotional and physical issues. Women especially hold on to this hurt in their centers, their wombs. All life comes from the womb. Afrikan nations depend on the womb to build and grow. Men have spiritual wombs too. Men and women have many relationship issues due to a myriad of factors. Afrikan women have forgotten what it was like to hold the Afrikan man in her womb, sending him love, protection, and healing. The Afrikan man has forgotten the womb from which he came. He has essentially forgotten who his mother is. He has forgotten floating in those sweet peaceful waters. Afrikan men and women were connected through the womb, vibrating on the same degree. This connection established harmony. They both have forgotten about the womb experience. The subconscious mind remembers the experience. Afrikans must go within and reclaim it. The womb is attacked through household chemicals, foods, and emotional issues. The emotional factor is a big component. Water carries emotions. Emotions alone can change the conditions of the womb including the taste of the amniotic fluid. Not only are Afrikans in a dire need of healing, but it must start in the primordial waters.

Afrikan women and men have to listen to the ancestor's advice. They are spiritual people with a connection to the universe. The people and the universe are one. The universe provides everything to heal thyself. Afrikans must live in a state of Maat. The netert (goddess) Maat teaches balance, truth, and reciprocity. The universe is composed of five elements: air, fire, water, earth, and ether. When these elements are balanced the body's mental, physical, and emotional health are balanced too. The elements can be related to traditional Afrikan herbal medicine. The pot contains water and the earth (herbs). Fire burns at the bottom of the pot. Hot air rises. The ether is the spirit of the Neteru/Orishas/Abosom/Loa (Afrikan deities), or the connection to the spirit which is omnipotent and in everything. This is taking the whole of what Afrikans have been given to heal the whole being including the divine spirit. Western medicine creates the illusion of healing. It does not address the whole being. Afrikans are whole people recognizing their connection to the whole of the universe. They see god in everything and every being. The Western world calls this paganism due to linear thought.

The ether element is associated with the ear and mouth. How did the beloved ancestors know which plants would heal? My guess is the ether element. Many people will say that a plant must be talked to if it is to grow properly. Some do not think about communing with the plant's spirit to help heal. Commune with the herbs, smell them, taste them, feel their texture, and absorb their color. See which herbs resonate with you. Take time to meditate on your situation and the plant. George Washington Carver was an excellent scientist and botanist because of his psychic ability to communicate with plant energy. His brother Jim, in watching George gently tending roses, once asked what he was doing. The boy's reply was that he was 'loving the flowers'.[1]

When I made my son's baby food I made it with love. I once blended some spinach for him when he was eleven-months-old. The green just sparkled like dark emeralds. I was at peace knowing that my son would be blessed that day with healing that would penetrate his whole being, his soul. I am so grateful to be his healer and grateful to the spirit for guiding me. Afrikans should consume things that heal the whole. Their actions should be beneficial to the elements. Are your actions devitalizing the air, water, and earth? Are your actions disconnecting you from the ether element that connects you to the spirit? Be mindful of what you eat and the products you use. Commercial cleaning products alone pollute the earth. Diapers sit in landfills when cloth diapering is available. On the Afrikan continent diapering is not needed. Parents in tune with their children are aware of when they need to eliminate. There is a multitude of ways traditional Afrikan lifestyle can improve homes and society.

1 - The Womb

The womb is the primordial waters from which all life comes from. The netert (goddess) Nu represents these waters. Ra, the life force, is the fire element which rose from the water element. His children are Shu and Tefnut, air elements. Shu and Tefnut gave birth to Geb, the earth element. Afrikan spirituality reflects the cosmology of the universe. The watery womb created the Neteru. Neteru is the name for the Khemetic (Ancient Nubian Egyptian) deities. Ask yourself, "Is my womb suitable for bringing forth the next gods who will walk this earth? Am I using the elements of the universe to create and heal?"

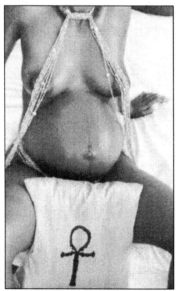

Courtesy of Kameela Abdul-Maajid,
Photography by Ava Griffith

The Afrikan woman's womb is attacked by hormonal birth control, pesticides, and toxins, just to name a few. Women also have womb issues related to holding on to hurt and pain. They sometimes curl their bodies up into a fetal position with their legs and arms close to the womb. Women take the hurt and give it to the womb. She will never be healthy if the womb center is holding pain and baggage. Women cannot bring forth healthy

11

children if they have been created in a womb that is dysfunctional. The mother and father must cleanse the whole being before conception. Once the child is conceived parents must begin nurturing the child while in the womb. Mother and father need to send the child loving and healing light daily. Parents must be conscious of the energy being sent. They should send only the divine and positive. The child is encapsulated in water. Water carries emotions. The baby can receive both positive and negative energy. Whether the mother is feeling joy, anger, or sadness the unborn child will feel it too. She has the ability to hear around 4 1/2 months. This is when the ear becomes functional. Iyas (mamas) sing Afrikan cultural songs to your babies and read to them in the womb. Babas (fathers) the child can hear your voice too. While, there is some evidence that the child hears the father's voice and that his voice has a calming affect on the newborn, the link between the child's ear and the father's voice is not even remotely as direct as the mother's voice. So, the greatest contribution that the expectant father can make is to love his child's mother.[1] In Senegal and Mali the father takes his special bond seriously, a father may loosen his belt during the mother's pregnancy to help establish his connection with the child. Sometimes during the mother's labor, the father will have his belt loosely wrapped around the mother's waist as an offering of his own nyama and support for the child's entry into the world.[2] Nyama is the life force. There is also evidence that the death of the father affects the unborn child. Researchers followed 167 children whose fathers had died before they were born, and 167 children whose fathers died during the first year of life. All 334 children grew up with no fathers present. However, only those who lost their father while in the womb were at increased risk of mental diseases, alcoholism, or criminality. [3]

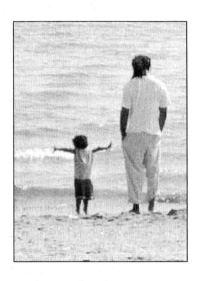

It is obvious that unborn children have an outside connection even while in the womb. Kings love your queens. Hold them up to the most high. Rub their feet and back. Help out with the cooking and cleaning around the house. Make her feel special. Prepare her an herbal bath. Take time out each day to show her your appreciation. Send her love, so that she may pass this love on to the child. Sending love to the womb is essential because so many toxic energies are present. The Environmental Working Group put out a report stating that unborn babies were stewing in a toxic soup. Ten samples of umbilical cord blood where taken from the Red Cross. They found an average of 287 contaminants in the blood, including mercury, fire retardants, pesticides, and the Teflon chemical PFOA. Also found were polyaromatic hydrocarbons, or PAHs, which are produced by burning gasoline and garbage, which may cause cancer; flame-retardant chemicals called polybrominated dibenzodioxins and furans; and pesticides including DDT and chlordane.[4] Mercury can damage the fetal brain and nervous system. Polyaromatic hydrocarbons increase the risk of cancer. Pesticides can cause fetal death and birth defects. Flame-retardant chemicals can hinder brain development. Some European countries have taken notice and are beginning to use less flame retardants. The United States, however, has not taken heed. The same group analyzed the breast milk of mothers across the United States in 2003 and found varying levels of chemicals, including flame retardants known as PBDEs.[4] The bedding many pregnant mothers and children sleep on contains flame retardants and toxic dyes. Tricia Edwards in the magazine *Black Woman and Child* states:

> Scientists have linked the chemicals to learning and memory impairment, thyroid deficiency, delayed puberty onset, behavioral imbalances, hearing loss, and fetal malformations. These toxins are much more detrimental to children. The organic industry offers many solutions. Mattresses can be made of certified organic cotton, pure wool, or a combination of the two. Avoid metal springs and the effects of Electromagnetic Radiation (EMR). The most common sources of EMR are high tension power lines, house wiring, household appliances, and mattress springs.[5]

Mothers can do many things to keep their babies safe in the womb. The universe balances negative and positive energy. Mothers can counter effect the negative energy with the following positive energy:

- Be peaceful, surround yourself with peaceful energies.
- Keep your surroundings in divine order, so you are in divine order.
- Refrain from gossip.
- Meditate, send healing light, energy, and colors to the womb.
- Eat as many organic fruits and vegetables as possible.
- If you are not a vegan, eat meat and dairy that is organic, hormone, and antibiotic-free if possible.
- Stay away from food that comes from the ocean. Unfortunately, the oceans are highly polluted with mercury.
- Avoid exterminators coming into the home; use other options such as boric acid for fleas and roaches. Pure peppermint oil keeps mice away.
- Avoid non-natural air fresheners.

14

- Use only natural home cleaning products; avoid chemicals such as Scotchgard in your home. Scotchguard is highly toxic.
- Use all natural personal body care.
- Avoid chemical relaxers, perms, and texturizers.
- Eat foods which are natural antioxidants to combat toxins.
- Avoid constant television watching and music that is not conducive to healing.
- Protect yourself from EMFs (electro-magnetic energy fields) and ELFs (low frequency electromagnetic energy fields) caused by: kitchen appliances, cell phones, televisions, microwaves, etc. Crystals such as black tourmaline, fluorite, and clear quartz can be used to combat harmful energy fields. Diodes can also be used to avoid EMFs and ELFs.
- Avoid lipsticks with lead.
- Avoid nail polishes with formaldehyde and phthalates. Water based nail polishes are available.
- Sleep on organic mattresses.

Crystal healing for pregnant mothers is recommended for deterring negative energy and improving overall health. The great ancestors of Khemit (Egypt) left the valuable tradition of crystal healing. Crystal healing can be used in all aspects of life especially childbirth, labor, and balancing children's energy. Pregnant women can carry medicine bags with crystals. However, medicine bags are not limited to the crystals. Mothers can carry the materials that are meaningful and sacred to their pregnancy such as words of power, tinctures, oils, cowries, and herbs. Great crystals for pregnant mothers to carry in their medicine bag are:

Rose Quartz
Rose Quartz can be used to send unconditional love to the baby.

Moonstone

15

Moonstone is a calming stone which can be used to balance the mother's emotions. Moonstone works with feminine energy and can make childbirth easier.

Malachite
Malachite protects against negative energy during pregnancy.

Unakite
Ukanite promotes healthy pregnancy and easy childbirth. It also supports the reproductive system.

Clear Quartz
Clear Quartz is an excellent universal healing stone. It generates energy and combats negative energy for all situations, including pregnancy.

These stones can also be worn as jewelry.

Vegan Diet during Pregnancy

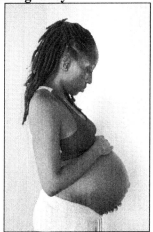

Courtesy of Kameela Abdul-Maajid,
Photography by Rory Dunn

A proper vegan diet is safe during pregnancy and lactation. Vegans do not eat the flesh of animals. Nor, do they eat animal by–products, such as milk and eggs. Many animals are pumped with antibiotics and hormones which are passed on to the womb.

16

Dead animal flesh and its by-products also carry adrenaline and poison. Adrenaline is produced when the animal experiences fear right before its death. This poison is not healthy for the unborn child. Dairy can be problematic also because it creates mucus. Mucus causes disease, tumors, and cysts. Milk also contains pus (white blood cells) and bacteria. A mother's caloric needs rise during pregnancy. According to Dr. McDougall, mothers will need 200 to 250 calories more a day. However, physically hard-working pregnant women from the Philippines and rural Africa take in no more, and often fewer calories, than before pregnancy. Fortunately, their foods are primarily nutrient-dense vegetable foods which will easily provide the raw materials to grow a healthy baby.[6] Afrikans are able to eat fewer foods, but eat foods consisting of more vegetables, and still provide for their babies. There is great value in plant based diets. Mothers do not need to consume large amounts of animal protein for a healthy and fit pregnancy.

I was successful maintaining a vegan diet during my pregnancy and lactation period. I know the vegan diet was vital in creating a smooth pregnancy. However, mothers should not change their diet drastically during pregnancy. This will result in the body rapidly detoxing. These toxins can be released to the baby. Vegan mothers concerned with whether or not they are eating correctly should consult a vegan nutritionist. They can provide nutritional counseling and can answer questions related to weight gain, caloric intake, fats, minerals, and vitamins needed.

When I was pregnant I was told I was anemic. I did not believe I was truly anemic and felt great. My midwife suggested that I take a popular herbal supplement that helps to make most people's hemoglobin counts rise. However, my count did not rise. She then suggested the herb yellow dock. Yellow dock did not work either. I also drank a lot of chlorophyll and added blackstrap molasses to my non-dairy milks. My midwife then suggested that my hemoglobin count may be what is normal for me.

Hemoglobin tests are not always effective, this test cannot diagnose iron deficiency, because the blood volume of pregnant women is supposed to increase dramatically, so the hemoglobin concentration indicates first the degree of blood dilution, an effect of placental activity...The regrettable consequence of routine evaluation of hemoglobin concentration is that, all over the world, millions of pregnant women are wrongly told that they are anemic and are given iron supplements.[7]

I did not abandon my vegan diet. I continued with my diet of fruits, vegetables, and whole grains. I made sure I ate a good helping of live foods daily. Fruit kept my stomach at ease and helped me to avoid morning sickness. My lunch always included raw, green, leafy vegetables. They contain many nutrients including vitamin A, vitamin C, calcium, and fiber. To keep my good fat intake up I ate a lot of avocados and added liquid vegetarian omega 3 6 9 fatty acids to my meals. Many vegans worry about B12. I am sure for some vegan mothers this worry may escalate. Most vegan mothers rely on B12 supplements, fortified foods, fermented foods, and nutritional yeast. Do not rely on nutritional yeast alone. A good multi-vitamin is ideal. The soil foods are grown in is sometimes depleted of nutrients.

Nutritional Chart

Vitamin A	Dark green leafy vegetables, carrots, sweet potatoes, broccoli, cabbage
Vitamin B 12	Nutritional yeast, Sublingual B-12 supplements, fortified foods
Vitamin B 1	Whole grains, brown rice, navy beans, kidney beans, oats, nuts, seeds, wheat germ
Vitamin B2	Green leafy vegetables and nuts
Vitamin B 6	Raw fruits, plantain, bananas, hazel nuts, spinach, potatoes
Vitamin B 9	Beans, whole grains, legumes, dark leafy vegetables
Vitamin C	Broccoli, oranges, papaya, guava, tangerines, kale, collard greens, kiwi
Vitamin D	Sunlight, torula yeast, fortified foods
Vitamin E	Wheat germ, spinach, broccoli,

	kiwi, almonds, green leafy vegetables, sweet potato
Vitamin K	Alfalfa, parsley, spinach
Protein	Nuts, beans, tofu, potatoes, wheat germ, oatmeal, kelp, duce, Irish moss, nori and spirulina
Iron	Blackstrap molasses, yellow dock, alfalfa, nettle, figs, watermelon, raisins, dark leafy green vegetables (kale, collards, spinach, etc.)
Omega 6	Safflower oil, sunflower oil, vegetables, fruits, nuts, whole grains, soybean
Omega 3	Spirulina, flax seeds, green leafy vegetables, hemp seed, pumpkin seed, avocado
Omega 9	Avocados, peanuts, olive oil, sesame seeds, peanuts, pecans, cashew, macadamia nuts
Calcium	Kale, collard greens, okra, Blackstrap molasses, tofu, broccoli, oatmeal, parsley

Meditation
There is a Malawi Chewa proverb that says, "Mother is god number two". Afrikan women are divine earth mothers who have been blessed with the ability to create. She is a Mut (moot), mother goddess. Afrikan mothers sit proudly on your throne, your seat. The name Auset means seat or throne. This great Netert (Khemetic goddess) was the ultimate mother. She was devoted to motherhood and marriage. Auset was a healer who brought her husband back to life. She is the mother who birthed a divine son who would bring order and righteousness to the world again. Auset lives within us all. Afrikan mothers must have the confidence to birth in their own images. The birth experience will be remembered for the rest of the mother's life, so it must be made a blessed event. Mothers are in control of their births and bodies. No one should interpret what the birth should be for the mother.

This is her blessed experience. The divine spirit manifesting in the womb should be protected. The same way Auset protected her son Heru from Set. Mothers have the right to question and say no.

Mothers can begin meditating on the birth as soon as they are aware that conception has taken place. She must prepare her body, mind, and spirit for a celestial birth. I visualized and meditated during my pregnancy. I sat in my bath tub of salt water. I talked to my son, guided him through our birth experience which was soon to come. I reassured him that it would be safe to leave the womb when it was time. I visualized him leaving my womb in a peaceful manner. I visualized my cervix opening slowly like a lotus flower, allowing his head to enter the birth canal. I envisioned him crowning slowly, and then pulling him up with my own hands onto my belly. I also sent healing colors and light to my womb. I massaged my womb. I let Yemaya (water) caress my womb. While in the bath I read the book, *Coming Forth by Day* to my son. *Coming Forth by Day,* also known as *The Egyptian Book of the Dead,* is one of the world's oldest books. It is essential that babies are exposed to enlightening literature. Music is also important; choose music such as Nina Simone, Sun Ra, John Coltrane, Pharaoh Sanders, and The Wailers, etc. Give your baby music and words that shine a healing light on the womb. Sit still, be at peace, and find your center. Take time to imagine your birth and what you need to do to create this heaven.

Altar work can also be used as a tool to connect with the baby. My altar included candles, a Yemaya doll, sea shells, plants, water, blue cloth, and crystals. The altar was centered around the Yoruba orisha Yemaya, mother of the orishas. She is the protector of mothers and their babies. Parents can create any type of altar that resonates with them and their baby's spirit. My altar was the special place where my baby and I could connect with each other. The women of the Dagara culture create shrines for their unborn babies. Thus, a shrine is, and will be, a sacred space that holds the baby's identity. Each time parents need to strengthen their bond with the baby or each other, they can return to the shrine.[8] The Dagara shrines consist of things such as plants, water, food, and medicine bags. Pregnant mothers should not underestimate the power of bonding with their babies through the womb. Mother and baby are literally one, complete harmony. The parents have the power to tune into their unborn child's needs. They must find a quiet and still place to communicate with their baby. Parents may ask the child if there is anything that she needs. Some ask the child why they have been so divinely chosen to be that child's parent. Parents may also choose to find out the child's destiny or life path. They should communicate daily. So, when the child comes to the earthly realm the parents and the child are in tune. This will enable them to meet their baby's needs and be on the same accord.

Preparation
Mothers can prepare their bodies physically. Some women prepare the perineum for birth to avoid tears. Commonly, oil is rubbed on the area to increase its elasticity. The Buganda women of Uganda sat in shallow baths of herbal preparations during the last few weeks of pregnancy to relax the tissues of the perineum. In nearby Sudan, the women would squat over a pot of herbs on the fire; this form of steaming moistened and softened the perineum and was held in great repute for making labours easier.[9]

The community can help the mother prepare for the birth also. Everyone is responsible for respecting and honoring the mother's queendom. Within the Afrikan community rituals are usually done for the mother and baby. Every Afrikan mother and child should have a blessing way. A blessing way is a rite of passage ceremony for the expectant mother. Blessing Ways usually has only females in attendance, including the doula and midwife. Men are sometimes in another room drumming. In Somalia, a ceremony takes place when the mother is 8-9 months pregnant. Only women are invited. Food and beverage are served and prayer takes place. The mother is also pampered, "We will put some oil in her hair. Then everybody massage around the stomach, massages the muscles there".[10] The Dagara culture also has rituals for the mother–to–be:

> A shrine is created for the baby during this ritual to facilitate communication between the parents and the child. The shrine usually starts with a gift of a medicine bag the grandparents bring to the ritual. Water, earth, plants, and fabrics are used to

21

create the shrine; the shrine can also contain precious items that others at the ritual may have brought for the mother-to-be and the baby. Contents of the shrine and the medicine bag increases as the parents - to- be are guided to bring items the incoming soul will point out to them during the duration of the pregnancy.[8]

Blessing Way Ideas

- Begin the ceremony by opening the way with libation to the ancestors.
- If possible have a traditional Afrikan priestess attend. The priestess can call on deities and ancestors. She can give divine information regarding the child's destiny, mission and much more.
- Each sista should be smudged with sage, myrrh, and frankincense.

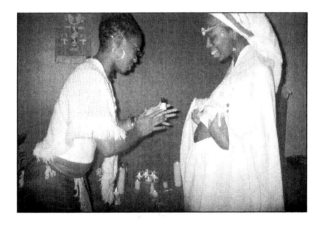

- Set up an altar for mother and baby. Use colors such as blue and white to represent mother deities such as Nu, Yemaya, and Auset. Place fresh flowers, plants, stones, crystals, and candles on the altar. Have guests bring altar gifts for mother and baby such as stones, poems, shells, and flowers. As each guest places their gift on the altar, they will explain its significance.

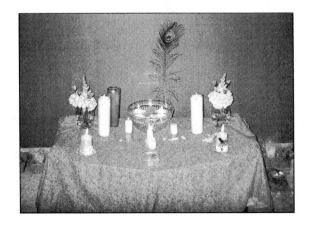

- Each sista should introduce themselves beginning with the mother – to – be by lighting a candle and stating, "I am "_____", daughter of "_____".The mother-to-be will light the next person's candle. This will create a lighted cipher of unity.

- A foot bath can be prepared for the mother-to-be with herbs and oils. While one of the sistas gives the mother a foot bath, the others can write words of inspiration in a journal for the mother-to-be.

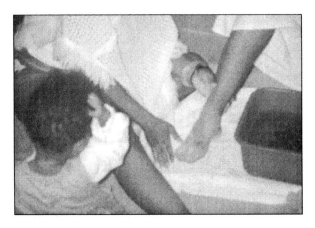

- Write down on pieces of paper fears concerning birth and motherhood. Burn the fears away in a fire–proof incense burner or holder; use charcoal and sage. The paper can be smudged with frankincense and myrrh.

- The ritual should be followed with a celebratory meal.

2 - Know Your Options & Your Rights

Choosing an Obstetrician and Gynecologist, Midwife, or Unassisted Birth

Parents can choose a midwife or an OB-GYN to deliver their baby. They can also choose to have their birth unassisted.

Midwives

The midwife is the original health care provider for all women. The traditional midwife mothered the mother-to-be. She helped her give birth in a respectable and honorable way:

> Early midwifery was characterized by spirituality, tradition, culture, and apprenticeship. Midwifery was passed down from mother to daughter. For many of the midwives, who often were not paid for their work, birthing babies was God's work and something that was done for the sake of the community and not money. Most importantly, Black midwives were holistic in their approach, often walking for miles to deliver babies and returning afterwards to make sure that the mother had food and to help the new mother care for younger children. Black Midwives kept alive African-based birth rituals such as the burial of the placenta, keeping a fire burning in the days following a birth, sweeping the house, smoking the house with cornmeal and walking the baby around the house saying the Lord's Prayer. Black midwives also used herbs and other natural remedies. The new mother also enjoyed a month-long rest after birthing, something that is sorely missing from the lives of new moms today. They did all this despite on-going assaults and condemnations from the medical establishment. As recently as 1950, Black midwives cared for as many as 50 percent of all Black babies born in some southern states.[1]

The calling to be a midwife was taken very seriously. Most Black midwives were not formally trained. Even when formally trained, many midwives believed that god guided them through the labor process. The wages were very low. Some midwives were paid in goods or food. There were also times when the family was so poor, the midwife fed the other children and made an outfit for the newborn baby to wear; because all some parents had for their newborn to wear was a blanket. Midwifery supplies were often very simple consisting of scissors, a piece of cloth to tie the umbilical cord, and herbs. Herbs were very important during the birth and labor process, unlike today. Some midwives were not under the supervision of doctors and could use the remedies of their choice. Grand midwife Onnie Lee Hogan states:

> In those days the doctors didn't tell em what to do. They used the old home remedies, mostly came from the Indian remedies. The midwife then would always carry her herbs that she was going to make teas out of to give them somethin warm to drink...There's a bush in the woods called the sassafras and you dig the root out of it. I love it.[2]

There are different types of midwives:

- Certified Nurse-Midwife (CNM) – She is trained in both nursing and midwifery. A bachelor's degree is required as well as certification from the American College of Nurse-Midwives. They are licensed to provide hospital, home, and birth center births. However, most provide hospital births.

- Certified Midwife (CM) – She has midwifery training and is not required to have nursing training. She is certified by the American College of Nurse Midwives.

- Certified Professional Midwife (CPM) – A professional midwife that has been certified by the North American Registry of Midwives.

- Lay Midwife – A midwife who chooses not to become certified or licensed. Their training is usually through apprenticeship or self study.

Unassisted
An unassisted birth is without the presence of a nurse, midwife, or OB-GYN. Some families choose this option because they find the presence of a midwife or OB-GYN simply unnecessary. Other women may not be able to have midwife attend their home births.

26

Many health insurance companies do not have many home birth midwives in their network or simply do not cover home births at all. A woman who chooses an unassisted birth relies on her earth mother instincts. She determines when its time to push instinctually or she may have her mate or attendee check dilation. Women who have children unassisted should not go to the hospital to get a birth certificate. Contact your state's department of vital records or town clerk. Hospitals cannot provide a birth certificate.

Some women who have unassisted births also do their own prenatal healthcare. They may purchase their on fetoscope, blood pressure monitor, and urine sticks to test protein in the urine. Fundal height is measured with measuring tape. It measures the area between the pelvis and upper uterus. The mother or her husband can check the baby's position with their hands. Many may think self prenatal care is dangerous, but studies have shown prenatal care has not been demonstrated to improve birth outcomes conclusively.[3] Dr. Michael Odent's assessment of prenatal visits:

> In many countries about ten prenatal visits are routine. In other words, most women have ten opportunities to hear about potential problems. At each visit a battery of tests is offered. These traditional patterns of medical care are based on the belief that the more antennal visits mean better outcomes. They have not based this on scientific data. [4]

Most women will not leave the OB-GYN's or CNM's office with a perfect bill of health. Many will leave scared, frustrated, or upset due to their tests results. This leads to stress which can cause poor health for mother and child. It is rare for a medical professional to find absolutely nothing wrong because of the large number of tests and their inaccuracies. The mother and father can decide which tests are important and which are not.

Obstetricians and Gynecologists (OB/GYN)
An Obstetrician and Gynecologist is a physician specializing in the reproductive system, pregnancy, and childbirth. Medical school and an OB/GYN residency program are required. OB/GYNs are certified by American Board of Obstetrics and

27

Gynecology. OB/GYNs attend hospital births. High risk mothers are recommended to seek their care.

Home, Birth center, or Hospital

Home birth

Home birthing is the traditional method of giving birth. During the middle ages in Europe, midwives faced persecution and were accused of being witches. Slowly, male physicians began to replace the midwives. Between 1910 and 1920 male physicians began to dominate midwifery in the United States. Midwifery was outlawed in many places. Today, more women are choosing midwives to deliver their babies in the home. Midwifery is still common in Afrika.

Home birth was the method of labor I chose to have because I wanted the most holistic birth possible. I had two midwives and a doula. My mate and the trinity composed of my mother, grandmother, and godmother attended the birth. Things fall in divine order when you let them and listen to the spirit. I never looked at the symbology of all three of my mothers helping to create a new trinity, mother, father, and son. The day of my son's birth I went to see my midwife and later went to work. After work I went to the market and a restaurant to eat. I arrived home in the evening around 7:30 P.M. By 8:30 P.M. my water had broken. I ran around all day. So, I had no rest. My midwife encouraged me to not work to late into the pregnancy. She warned me that I would not have ample rest for labor. She was right. My son was posterior and my placenta was anterior. Posterior is when a baby is facing sunny side up. The position is not ideal. An anterior placenta is when the placenta is in front of the baby. Placentas usually are above the baby. These positionings caused my water to break first. Hard labor came quickly. I was in a lot of pain. Within twenty minutes all my water bags broke. I found that I could not lie down at all. My contractions were most bearable when sitting on the toilet. I was in an ideal squatting position with the gravity of water assisting me. Water is symbolic of Yemaya/Auset. So, my body was able to relax a lot more. I also had in my bathroom incense and crystals. My crystal were clear quartz, rose quartz, and malachite. I listened to one of Ra Un

28

Nefer Amen's Auset devotion meditation CDs. The chants assisted me in my meditation. Auset had sorrows and pains, but her devotion got her through trying times and she was able to birth a new light, Heru! So I kept this in mind and let her spirit guide me. I also sat down in the shower and just let the water run over my body. The spirit ran over me. I needed to connect with my mothers Het Heru, Oshun, Yemaya, Auset, Meshkenet, and Nana Esi Ketewaa. I did connect with the goddesses. I was able to stay focused because of the spirit. I had a very painful labor. I did not have much space between contractions. I had an inflatable pool that was being filled up while I waited in the bath tub. But my cat fell in the pool and ripped holes into it. So, the pool was drained cleaned and re-filled. I actually did not labor long in the water. Water birth is usually very beneficial for mothers. This was not the case for me. I actually labored on my bed. I had a cervical lip that would not budge. So I decided to get out of the water. My midwife offered me assistance by holding the lip back while I pushed. Finally, my son was delivered while I was on all fours. The labor was thirteen hours total. My birth was long and painful. However, it was perfect. I wouldn't change a thing about my birth. I have no regrets. It was my birth, a birth I dictated. I was in control and allowed to be the divine mother creator I was destined to be.

After the birth, my legs were cramped from being in one position for a long period of time while I was pushing. My midwife gave me the herb arnica to relieve the stiffness. After I had time to bond with my baby, she dressed him just as a traditional midwife would do. My midwife was aware of where the baby's clothes, chuck pads, and other birth supplies were, because she made a visit to my home to help me prepare for the birth. The experience was very personal. Midwife Onnie Lee Hogan testifies about being prepared:

> I meet all my patients for three to fo' different times when they engage me befo' I deliver that baby. Rules and regulations were that we were supposed to make those pads and have things ready for that mother befo' the time of delivery. Myself and the mother together made the pads at her house. Do not wait until the exact time or the week befo'. Make preparations. Go and

visit em. Talk with em. Look at the bed. See how the bed's set up cause I can't work left-handed.[2]

My midwife was wonderful. Before leaving my home, she made sure I had something to eat and was comfortable. She confined me to the second floor of my house for two weeks.

Women experiencing natural labor travel to another place. They go within and center themselves. Women go into a primitive state where they lose many inhibitions. During my own labor I could care less about my family seeing me naked or hearing me make strange noises. Prior to my birth I had no idea why women lost inhibitions. The neocortex causes women to become inhibited. Such inhibitions originate in the 'new brain', the part of the brain that is highly developed among humans and which can be seen as the brain of the intellect, or thinking brain. It leads us to understand that a labouring woman needs first to be protected from any sort of stimulation of the neocortex.[4] Suppressing neocortex activity makes the labor process easier. Many factors can stimulate the neocortex, bright lights, little privacy, and insecurity.

During a study women planning home births were matched with women having hospital births. Studies revealed the following findings for the home birth group:

> There were fewer interventions during labour, including electronic fetal monitoring, induction of labour, episiotomy, and cesarean section; women were more likely to have an intact perineum and fewer maternal infections and were no more likely to have third-degree or fourth-degree tears or postpartum hemorrhage; and there were no significant differences in perinatal mortality, 5-minute apgar scores and meconium aspiration syndrome, as compared with women intending to deliver in hospital who were assisted by physicians or midwives.[5]

Many people believe home births are not safe because the home is not sterile. Since the newborn baby has the same levels of such antibodies as its mother, this implies that the microbes that are familiar to the mother are also familiar to the germ-free newborn

30

baby.[4] The actual location of birth can affect mother and child. Psychiatrist Ryoko Hattori found children born in a particular hospital had higher rates of autism. In that particular hospital the routine was to induce labor a week before the expected date of birth and to use a complex mixture of sedatives, anesthesia agents and analgesics during labor. [4]

Hospital Births

Some women prefer OB-GYNs over midwives. There are cases when an OB-GYN is better suited to deliver a baby. However, many healthy Afrikan women have a better chance for a safe and fulfilling birth at home or at a birth center. Families choosing hospital births must know their rights. If there are certain things the family wants or does not want they must be firm and persistent. Any sign of weakness can give way to a birth that is over medicated or not as planned. As a doula who has attended hospital births I have seen with my own eyes how easily a mother and father can be persuaded with fear. Having a good birth plan your doctor is aware of ahead of time is essential. Parents must always emphasize to the ob/gyn on each visit what type of birth they want. Parents should choose a physician or midwife that is encouraging and has the same birth and labor philosophies. They should also ask them about their c-section and episiotomy rates.

Key Things Parents Should Know:
- IVs are not always necessary. They hamper movement. Heparin locks are available. Or mothers can simply drink juices to provide hydration instead of an IV.
- Laboring on the back is not necessary. Families can bring their own birthing ball or squatting chair. Make use of the furniture in the room along with the toilet.
- Placentas can be kept. To accomplish this, families must be firm and persistent. As soon as the staff is done examining the placenta have a container ready and tell them to place your placenta in it. Do not let them take your placenta out the room; it is highly unlikely you will get it back.
- Antibiotics placed in the child's eyes can be waived as well as the vitamin K shot. Antibiotics are only

31

needed for mothers who have gonorrhea and chlamydia. Oral vitamin K is available for families who prefer not to give their children the vitamin K injection.

- The Hepatitis B vaccine can be refused.
- Healthy babies do not have to leave the room. If families are confronted with hospital staff who want to remove a healthy baby from the presence of both parents, ask to see a superior.
- Newborn baths can be refused.

The baby should be breastfed immediately after birth. Parents who have hospital deliveries should request time with their baby before routine procedures if the child is healthy. Avoid unnecessary poking and prodding. Request the umbilical cord blood be used to identify the baby's blood type. Because, I had a home birth I was able to sign a phenylketonuria (PKU) test waiver to opt out. This tests screens for other metabolic disorders other than PKU such as hypothyroidism and cystic fibrosis. Some parents do not want the test performed on their child. Opting out may be more difficult in a hospital setting if you choose to waive the test. Some parents have issues with the tests accuracy. There is much controversy surrounding how accurate the test is and when it should be administered. The test is done by lancing the baby's foot with a heel stick to collect blood. Birth plans can make the hospital staff aware of the family's birth preferences ahead of time.

The Chidi's Birth Plan

The purpose of this birth plan is to provide the hospital staff with an understanding our philosophies concerning birth and labor. We look forward to a pleasant and uncomplicated birth. Our family has prepared for a natural birth, and would like to create an environment conducive to this goal. We would like a hospital birth with minimum medical intervention. However, we are aware complications may arise. If so, we would like informed consent of all procedures, giving us the chance to accept or refuse any procedure.

1. We would prefer a peaceful birth environment. We requests the lights be kept dim and the door closed. Please have only the minimum number of staff come into the room. We do not want any students or observers in the room.
2. Fluids for hydration are preferred instead of IV usage. If this is not an option we would like a heparin lock for mobility instead of an IV.
3. Do not offer epidurals or narcotics for pain relief.
4. We prefer to labor in the position of our choice.
5. We prefer not to have an episiotomy.
6. The cord is not to be cut until it stops pulsating and all nutrients are transferred.
7. We prefer to breastfeed our baby immediately after the birth.
8. We plan to breastfeed, please do not give our baby bottles, pacifiers, or water.
9. Do not give the Vitamin K shot to our child.
10. We do not want antibiotic ointment/drops placed in our baby's eyes after birth.
11. The child is to remain with the mother and father at all times.
12. We prefer our child not be bathed.

Birth Centers

Today, more parents are deciding to give birth at free-standing birth centers. They find the birth center more home-like than hospitals. Some parents find comfort in the fact that most birth centers are close to hospitals. Birth centers are more supportive of natural birth than hospitals. Good birth centers treat birth like a normal event. Many have a bedroom, family room, kitchen, dining room, and jacuzzi tub. CNMs (Certified Nurse Midwives) are the most common types of midwives at birth centers. The mother may stay at the birth center for 7-12 hours after birth. Some birth centers have narcotic analgesia on site that can be given to the mother if she wants them, but many birth centers try to avoid using narcotics.

Doulas
Doulas attend hospital, birth center, and home births. She will usually bring a doula bag which may contain, massage tools, lotions, oils, aromatherapy, and hot and cold packs. She also may take pictures, video, and notes for a birth story. Doulas can help parents achieve the birth they want in a hospital, birth center, or home environment. They can especially be a great advocate in a hospital environment. A doula is trained to provide labor support only. Doula is a Greek word meaning women care giver or woman's servant. A doula is a birth attendant or labor assistant that supports women during pregnancy, labor, and postpartum. This support addresses the family's physical and emotional needs. Doulas let parents know they have choices. A doula does not decide what is best for the family. But, supports the decisions they choose. They encourage women to find their voice at one of the most memorable times of their lives.

The benefits of having a doula:

- Less pain and stress during labor
- Decrease in caesarean rate
- Less postpartum depression
- Helps to bring the husband closer to mother during labor
- Can assist with a variety of labor positions
- Studies have shown, doulas help reduce unnecessary medical interventions and improve the health of mother and baby

Midwives

Why have so many of us forgotten how to give Birth?

We've been doing it since the beginning of our time on Earth

Our strengths were replaced by fears

By medicalizing birth through out the years

The power was taken away from the Midwives

They were the ones that protected Birth and saved many women and babies lives

The male order turned them into the image of a witch

Spreading propaganda; saying that they were the devils own bitch

They replaced the women squatting on stools

With doctors sitting on them giving their rules

We've been told for so long that In sorrow we shall bring forth life

Well, it doesn't have to be that way if you have a Midwife!

Doctors tried to leave Midwives without any power

They were afraid of a woman that could heal with herbs and barks even a flower!

My sisters please breastfeed!

Don't you want what is best for your seed?

I fed my babies past two and a half

Because they were never meant to drink milk that is for a calf

Peace on Earth Begins at Birth

Give Birth at home and not medicated

Because strong women they want obliterated

Remember your history but dont get stuck

You gotta live in the present cause most people dont give a F*@#k!

Make strong families and make them last

That's how you brake free from the chains of the past!

-Venus Paloma Rodriguez-McGregor

Venus Paloma Rodriguez-McGregor BS CD LCCE was born in San Juan, Puerto Rico and moved to NY when she was 8 years old. Venus is the mother of three beautiful children. She lives in Spring Valley, NY with her husband and children.

3 - OB/GYNs and the Medicalization of Childbirth

Prenatal Testing

Expectant mothers will be asked or urged to take many tests. Tests may include rubella antibodies, triple screen, anemia, Rh factor, gonorrhea, chlamydia, and sickle cell anemia. Parents have the right to refuse these tests. Parents will be asked if they would like to test for Down syndrome. However, this test is highly inaccurate and produces many false results. This can cause parents needless worrying. Parents can also make suggestions concerning testing. Gestational diabetes testing is pretty much routine. Most physicians will have the mother drink a carbonated glucose drink. A more healthy option, just as accurate is orange juice.

The test most concerning is the HIV test. Only New York and Connecticut have mandatory HIV testing for newborns. However, this can be avoided by home birth. In these two states, if the child is born in a hospital they will be tested without the mother and father's consent if the mother refused the test during prenatal visits. New Jersey is working to pass a law also, to have mandatory HIV testing for pregnant mothers and newborns. The problem with HIV tests are their accuracy. HIV tests do not test for HIV or AIDS. The test looks for reactive antibodies and proteins. The antibody test is not specific to HIV antibodies. The ELISA and Western blot tests use this method. The ELISA test serum must be diluted 400 times. The Western blot serum must be diluted 50 times. If the ELISA serum is not diluted the result is positive for every test. Dr. Roberto Giraldo states:

> The results presented here could also mean that the tests used for detecting antibodies to HIV are not specific for HIV, as has been explained previously. In this case, there would be reasons other than HIV infection, past or present, to explain why a person reacts positive to it. The test also reacts positive in the absence of HIV. The scientific literature has documented more than 70 different reasons for getting a positive reaction other than past or present infection with HIV. All these conditions have in common a history of polyantigenic stimulations...The only proper way for establishing the sensitivity and specificity

37

of a given test is with a gold standard. However, since HIV has never been isolated as an independent purified viral entity, there cannot be a gold standard for HIV.[1]

He also states that in the United States the ELISA and Western blot tests are done together. The Western blot antigens, proteins or bands which are considered to be specific to HIV, may not be encoded by the HIV genome and may in fact represent human cellular protein.[2]

The Polymerase Chain Reaction (PCR) viral load test is also used. It is not approved by the FDA to diagnosis HIV. Viral loads are found in those who tests positive and negative for HIV. Viral load tests detect and multiply only fragments of genes, not HIV. Tests manufactures warn that viral load cannot confirm the presence of HIV.[3] Nobel Laureate Dr. Kary Mullis who invented the Polymerase Chain Reaction test explains that "PCR makes it possible to identify a needle in a haystack by turning the needle into a haystack." While PCR has provided many realms of science and industry with an effective new tool, its application to AIDS research has been far more misleading than useful.[3]

Many factors can result in a false positive including hepatitis, flu, cold, HLA antibodies and pregnancy. There is also a higher rate for false positives among women who have had prior pregnancies. If a mother receives a false positive she has the potential of becoming sick emotionally and physically due to the test result. The results can cause depression and anxiety that can affect the overall health of baby and mother. Most doctors will prescribe retrovirals to HIV positive mothers which cause AIDS related illnesses such as anemia, pneumonia, and tubercolis. Contrary to popular belief, AIDS is not a new disease. AIDS is a new name given by the Center for Disease Control (CDC) to a collection of 29 familiar illnesses and conditions including yeast infection, herpes, diarrhea, some pneumonias, certain cancers, salmonella and tuberculosis.[3] These conditions have not always been fatal in the past, nor do they have to be now. These diseases can be acquired without having a positive HIV result. However, the medical industry equates HIV positive antibody tests with any of these conditions as AIDS.

Many retrovirals actually can cause AIDS related symptoms. Glaxo SmithKline's Retrovir prescription sheets states:

> Immune reconstitution syndrome has been reported in patients treated with combination antiretroviral therapy, including RETROVIR. During the initial phase of combination antiretroviral treatment, patients whose immune system responds may develop an inflammatory response to indolent or residual opportunistic infections (such as Mycobacterium avium infection, cytomegalovirus, Pneumocystis pneumonia [PCP], or tuberculosis), which may necessitate further evaluation and treatment.[4]

Some pregnant women who have used AZT had babies with severe birth defects and malformations. Unfortunately, HIV negative babies born to HIV positive mothers are treated with AZT for the first six months of their lives. Some of babies develop pneumocystic carini pneumonia. Pneumonia and tuberculosis are two diseases classified as AIDS. Retrovirals are also known to cause bone marrow loss. Retrovirals actually attack the immune system and causes AIDS related symptoms. Pregnant Afrikan mothers should research all diseases they are being tested for closely, especially HIV.

Ultrasounds

Many parents are excited to see images of their baby in the womb. But, before rushing to get ultrasounds their safety must be researched. Parents should know the risks of all procedures before exposing a fetus to high frequency sound waves. Energy enters the womb during the procedure. This energy affects fetal tissue, having thermal affects on fetal tissue, which changes its temperature. Most insurance companies only pay for one ultrasound for low-risk mothers. Today ultrasound studios provide parents with three and four dimensional pictures. These ultrasounds allow parents to see more than the 2D picture, but allow parents to actually see the baby's features. 3D ultrasounds are sometimes performed by unskilled technicians and are allowed to be done for non medical purposes, without consent from a physician. The 3D and 4D ultrasounds emit more energy than the standard 2D ultrasounds. Studies have shown exposure to ultrasounds does affect the fetus:

> Obstetric ultrasound examination is part of routine antenatal care and is regarded as safe for both the fetus and the mother. In vitro, however, ultrasound has been shown to cause membrane changes that could affect embryogenesis and late prenatal and postnatal development. Studies have also shown an association between exposure to ultrasound and an increased frequency of non-righthandness, indicating that fetal development may be affected by the ultrasonic waves.[5]

Other studies have shown premature babies are five times more likely than normal to be left-handed. According to the Swedish researchers, the human brain undergoes critical development until relatively late in pregnancy, making it vulnerable to damage. In addition, the male brain is especially at risk, as it continues to develop later than the female brain.[6] Healthy mothers who choose to get ultrasounds should limit them to one if possible and only get them from skilled professionals. Routine ultrasound scanning does not improve the outcome of pregnancy in terms of live births or of reduced perinatal morbidity. Routine ultrasound scanning may be effective and useful as a screening for malformation. Its uses for this purpose, however, should be made explicit and take into account the risk of false positive diagnosis in addition to the ethical issues.[7]

Chemical Inductions
Pitocin, cytotec, and cervidil are the most common methods used for chemical inductions.

Pitocin is the most commonly used. It is synthetic oxytocin. Oxytocin is the hormone produced during joy, laughter, and sex. The same oxytocin used to make the baby is needed to soften and ripen the cervix. Pitocin tries to mimic this. Natural oxytocin is the releasing of love hormones. This is the one reason among others to assume that a woman develops a certain extent her capacity to love while giving birth.[7] One of the major downsides of pitocin for mothers who want to have a birth without epidurals and narcotics is that it makes contractions unbearable. They are far worse than contractions without pitocin. Pain is also hard to endure when movement is hindered. Fetal monitoring is required as well as an IV, limiting mobility. Risks associated with pitocin are fetal malpresentation, caesarian, fetal distress, fetal heart rate problems, and uterine rupture.

Cervidil is a prostaglandin which can cause the cervix to ripen. The male's sperm is a natural prostaglandin. Cervidil is inserted in the mother's vagina for a period of time and then removed. Cervidil can cause uterine hyperstimulation.

Cytotec is another method of chemical induction. However, it is only FDA approved for usage as a drug for gastric ulcers. One of the dangers of cytotec is that unlike pitocin and cervidil, there is no standard dosage. The effects of cytotec cannot be slowed down or removed once given to the mother. Many hospitals are opting to use cytotec over pitocin and cervidil because it is fast-acting and cheap. Cytotec has been known to cause uterine rupture, uterine hyperstimulation, injury to mother, and amniotic fluid embolism which can result in death.

Narcotics
The narcotics used are Demoral, Stadol, Nubane, and Fentanyl. Narcotics are giving through an IV. They dull the pain, not take the pain away. Narcotics can depress the mothers breathing, affect fetal heart rate, the baby's blood ph, and interfere with its ability to suckle.

Epidurals
Epidurals are used to stop pain during labor. A needle is placed in the mother's back between the vertebraes. Unlike narcotics, the mother is completely aware and awake. The body is numb from the waist down, but the mother is able to feel some sensation. IV's and continuous electronic fetal monitoring are required. Bladder catheters are also used. Epidurals have been associated with slowing down labor, often leading to chemical inductions, and caesarean sections. Epidurals can affect the unborn child. The anesthesia does pass through the placenta. Babies can experience fetal distress. Some babies have breastfeeding latching trouble. Mothers sometimes experience chills and a drop in blood pressure. If the needle or the catheter migrates inward, convulsions,

41

respiratory paralysis, and/or cardiac arrest can occur. These latter two complications have been reported to occur as commonly as 1 in 3,000 cases.[8] Some women experience postpartum headache, back pain, and nerve damage.

Electronic Fetal Monitoring (EFM)
Consistent electronic fetal monitoring can sometimes be a hindrance for mothers wishing to labor naturally. EFM causes the mother to have to lie on her back. EFM is required if an epidural or chemical induction is being used. Many doctors believe EFM can recognize if the baby is getting insufficient oxygen, preventing mental retardation, death, or cerebral palsy. Author of *The Thinking Woman's Guide to a Better Birth*, Henci Goer states:

> Less than 10 percent of cases of cerebral palsy or mental retardation during or shortly after birth result from oxygen deprivation during labor." The number of cases of oxygen deprivation in labor has declined steeply since 1979. If birth asphyxia were largely responsible for cerebral palsy, the cerebral palsy rate should have declined too.[8]

Even though there is no real evidence consistent electronic fetal monitoring is valuable, doctors are reluctant to limit the use if it. It is less work for the medical team. Nurses can monitor the mother from the nurse's station and the EFM report can be used in malpractice suits. Intermittent fetal monitoring is a better option for low risk mothers. It will not confine the mother to labor on her back.

Episiotomy
Many doctors routinely give episiotomies to prevent the mother from tearing. An episiotomy is a surgical cut in the perineum area between the vagina and the anus. Medical studies have proven this procedure is unnecessary. It is a cruel and barbaric. The recovery period can be painful and there is a chance of infection. Many women are scared to move their bowels or urinate after the procedure due to fear. There are ways to prepare the perineum through massage and oil. The positions used during labor can also help. It has been found tears that naturally occur compared to

episiotomies heal faster. *The British Medical Journal* published an article, stating:

> The use of episiotomy is a paradigmatic example of the many interventions that are introduced into clinical practice without scientific evidence and found after well performed research to be not only unjustified but also possibly harmful. In addition, once an intervention has been established in clinical practice it is not easily abandoned, even when strong scientific evidence shows its uselessness and harmfulness.[9]

Caesarean

Caesarean section is a method of delivery. It is a horizontal cut along the bikini line, usually no more than four inches long. Caesarean section in the United States is increasingly becoming more common. It is the most common major surgical procedure performed in the Unites States.[8] Some women are electing to have the procedure. Many women are told by their physicians a caesarean is the best option. Physicians receive more money for caesareans. They are more convenient for some doctors. There are cases where caesareans are life saving for mother and baby. However, caesareans cause more maternal deaths than vaginal birth. A 1989 analysis in Great Britain revealed that women were 550 percent more likely to die of an elective caesarean than a vaginal birth.[8] Some cesarean born babies score low on their apgar scores. Caesareans can cause babies to be born in poor conditions. There is an accumulation of data confirming that, in general a caesarean born baby (particularly a baby born after a non-labour caesarean) is physiologically different from a baby born by the vaginal route. Let us comment also on the findings of an Italian study, according to which the amount of endorphins in the milk of the first days is much higher among mothers who gave birth vaginally compared with mothers who underwent caesarean section.[7] The caesarean recovery period can be very painful. The mother will need help attending to her needs as well as the baby's during the recovery period. Some mothers have trouble trying to heal from an operation and attend to a newborn.

A normal childbirth in a hospital can be a rare event. Parents must be educated and empowered. Birth is a natural event that does not always require a highly medicalized environment. The cold, metal, and "sterile" environment does not help. The room also has a lot of computers that emit electromagnetic fields. If parents are questioning whether a hospital birth is for them they should consider what Johanson and Newburn have found:

> There is evidence that obstetric interventions in labour tend to lead from one to another. Women who have labour induced need more help with pain relief, epidurals lead to more instrumental births, and perineal trauma causes dyspareunia. Long term morbidity after childbirth may be significant and is particularly related to instrumental and caesarean delivery. Specific concerns relate to painful intercourse and urinary and anal incontinence. Even elective caesarean section does not avoid these particular complications, which may have a closer relation to pregnancy itself than the mode of delivery. Doctors have a duty not to harm their patients, so must ensure that any care does more good than harm, taking into account long term as well as short term effects.[10]

Physical and Psychological Affects of an over medicalized birth

Many Afrikan children in the United States have asthma. Cow's milk has been associated with asthma. However, birth practices too can contribute to asthma. Studies have shown perinatal factors are associated with childhood asthma. The current analyses examined the association between obstetric complications and risk of asthma at the age of 7 years using a prospectively population-based birth cohort in northern Finland.[11] Studies have found that caesarean section, vacuum extraction, and the use of forceps are associated with asthma. The conditions children are born under can follow them for the rest of their lives. Many parents have no clue that birth conditions may have long term psychological consequences. Dr. Michael Odent has researched primal health extensively. He describes the primal period as fetal life, perinatal period, and early infancy, Odent states:

> Juvenile violent criminality is undoubtedly topical. It can be regarded as a form of an impaired capacity to love others. Adrian Raine and his team from the University of California in Los Angeles followed 4,269 male subjects born in the same hospital in Copenhagen. They found that the main risk factor for being a violent criminal at age 18 was the association of birth

44

complications, together with early birth separation from or rejection by the mother. Early maternal separation-rejection by itself was not a risk factor.[12]

Studies have also shown teenage suicide involving asphyxiation is more common with babies who had asphyxiation at birth. There is also evidence narcotics given to the mother at birth can increase the likelihood of her child being addicted to drugs as a teenager. Doctors Jacobson and Karin Nyberg looked at the background of 200 opiate addicts born in Stockholm from 1945 to 1966 and took non-addicted siblings as controls. They found if a mother had been given certain painkillers during labor, her child was statistically at an increased risk of becoming drug-addicted in adolescence.[12]

Hospital acquired infections are also becoming more common. Parents must be aware of antibiotic resistant infections. Hospitals have a lot of foot traffic and sick people. This is in direct contrast to the home, the environment to which mother and baby are accustomed. There is a small chance of such an infection in a birth center. The very young and elderly are especially susceptible to hospital infections.

Birth essays and poems from Iyas and Babas (Mothers and Fathers)

Melinda's Birth Story
By Melinda Blythe

I was determined not to sit in the sterile hospital bed pumped full of drugs and chemicals, made docile so that I could easily fit into the doctor's rotation. My child's entrance into this world would not be under the haze of narcotics or the jostling of hands plucking him from my shattered womb. He would be guided, pushed into the soft light by the same muscles that cradled him, nurtured and shielded him from the harshness of what was to come. He would be ready, and he would do his part, wriggling, tilting, and tucking his little head. This was the first step in making him aware of his own destiny. His role would not be overlooked, nor his will disregarded. So, I rejected the idea of introducing pitocin into my bloodstream. Especially not four times the FDA regulated amount I had been duped into getting during my first delivery. Why speed things along when my body was telling me what time it was? At 5:05 P.M. the night before, I started having regular contractions. By three in the morning I was doubled over feeling the burn and strain in my lower back and ileopsoas. My water had broken naturally by 7:20 A.M. and we decided it was time to head in.

Immediately I was placed on antibiotics for Group B strep; a condition that I am told afflicts many mothers these days. This limited my mobility. My child's heartbeat also had to be monitored constantly with a belly strap. For whatever reason, whenever I drew myself up to an upright position it sent his heart rate into flux. So, once again technology had me in an awkward position. I was laying flat in a hospital bed. I imagined how I wanted my delivery to be. I fantasized about a water birth in a warm pool of non chlorinated water, using a physio ball and birthing stool. All of those options had been readily dismissed upon my admission to the hospital. But I did have some degree of control over what I allowed into my body. Pitocin or any other drugs to speed the process were not making the cut. I relaxed into each contraction comforted by the knowledge that I was doing the

46

best I could to give my baby the best start in life. I reflected on the pregnancy and the many stages that I'd gone through. I remembered the total body swell that had me glowing from the inside out, the womanly curves that adorned my bones and filled my clothing with life. I contemplated on the pimples, hormonal roller coasters, cravings, fears, and uncertainties about becoming a parent again. I had a real fear about delivering a large being from my not so large vagina. One would think that by the time you were able to deliver you'd have come to grips with this, but on the contrary, the larger I got (and the baby) the more fearful I had become about my ability to have a successful VBAC (Vaginal Birth after Caesarean).

During the delivery I focused a lot on breathing. I mentally relaxed each muscle that wasn't directly responsible for releasing the baby. It was easy to tense everything up in pain. It took concentration to let it go and let my body do what it was intrinsically capable of, as countless women before me. I was joining the ranks in this rite of passage.

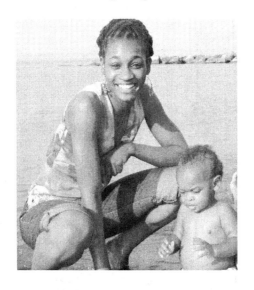

Courtesy of Melinda Blythe,

Photography by Laura Thompson

47

Melinda Blythe is a mother of three children: six-year-old Nailah Dara Phillips, Khaalida Ama (deceased,) and twenty-one-month Jelani Asad Phillips. She is also dancer, Co-founder of the dance company Ba Bes Dance, and a writer for the Written Raw Arts.

Cris' Birth Story

By Cris

I don't know where to begin. I've been a mom for 4 1/2 months now and I am still amazed. I look at my little Elijah Kahlil and feel this overwhelming amount of love that still shocks me. How did I get here? What led up to this pure bliss that I'm feeling? I think back to my pregnancy. My pregnancy was a healthy one, aside from a short period of emotional confusion. But, pregnancy attracts many different types of energies, whether they are wanted or not. Everyone had an opinion. These same people want to share horrid pregnancy and labor stories even if they've never been pregnant. I never had it in me to politely ask people to keep the negativity to themselves. They were simply sharing. How could I argue that? So I let them release and then politely countered their energy with what I was feeling or thinking, which was always positive concerning my pregnancy. I was excited to be creating life even during the first trimester when I felt physically ill and exhausted every single day. I took care of myself by eating well, exercising, and getting all of the sleep that my body requested. In the meantime, I read some incredible birthing stories such as Ina May Gaskin's *Spiritual Midwifery,* an incredible inspiration.

I had chosen to give light to my baby in my own home. Women didn't start using doctors until recently. Relatively speaking, ever since, the act of birth has gotten scarier for us. We have somehow forgotten that our bodies were MADE to do this. Our bodies work just fine. We don't need c-sections, vacuums, or forceps. Our babies don't need doctors to catch, suction, bathe, and wrap them up in cotton. Our babies need to be born into loving and comforting arms. Our babies need to feel skin and smell their moms instantly, moms need this too.

I had incredible midwives who validated me and made me feel safe about making such a natural choice. It is sad that we have come to a place where we question what is natural and blindly trust what is only been in existence for a century. During my pregnancy I was sure to keep my body and mind as healthy as possible. I continued to be physically active. I did yoga until only two weeks before I pushed Elijah out. I felt wonderful and I fully trusted my body. I met so many women who just wanted the baby out by the end of the seventh month. There wasn't a single moment when I felt that way. I was fortunate enough to not feel any notable discomforts until the last two weeks. But even with those discomforts I was happy to feel life within me. I knew that those discomforts meant something. It was okay. It was not going to be permanent. More than anything, it would be worth it. People would say funny things like, "You must be tired of being pregnant by now!" Why do people just assume this? I was always glad to let them know that every woman did not feel that way. I certainly didn't. I felt radiant, big belly, and all! I still felt quite agile, considering.

Then the day came. I woke up earlier than normal feeling a bit crampy. I knew the time was near. My body had been experiencing some different things over the last two weeks or so. Eric and I went about running errands and such. For the first time there were short little periods when I had to stop walking. Sounds obvious, but I had no idea I was in labor. After running our errands I took a three hour nap. I woke up and went to my chiropractic appointment and hung out with some friends. I skipped my usual yoga class, something I rarely did. I was just too tired. I had been planning a water birth; but the tub wasn't set up yet. Around 9 P.M., Eric and I decided we should get the tub set up given my due date was only ten days away. But then we decided to watch a movie instead. The movie ended at 11:30 P.M. As I laid in bed, trying to fall asleep, I realized that sleep was no where near. That's when I realized that I was in labor. I decided that at least one of us should sleep, so I left Eric and went into to living room to read. I got antsy after a while, so I tidied the house up and did some laundry. Yes, you read it correctly. Labor very rarely comes on the way that the media projects. The overall process is slow, preparing our bodies for the work, the labor that lies ahead. I left a voice message for my midwives at 2:30 A.M. I didn't want to disturb them knowing that I wasn't in active labor yet, so I just left a warning on the voice mail. At 3 A.M. I decided that I should at least lie down. I went to bed at 4 A.M. As I was getting up to pee my warm waters gushed all over the place. I giggled while Eric cleaned up and got me some dry clothes. He wanted to call the midwives immediately. I didn't think it was necessary yet. We agreed that Eric would first time the contractions just so that we had something concrete to say. It turned out my contractions were five minutes apart. This means that labor is kicking in for those unfamiliar with the process. So, Eric called one of the midwives, and while she was telling him to have me take a warm shower to relax my contractions began to kick in hard core. Hearing them, my midwife decided it was time to come on over.

Our midwives, childbirth education classes, and our readings taught us to prepare for a full days worth of labor. So, we were prepared to be up for the next twenty-four hours. Sure, I had been in labor all day, but I didn't even know it. So, although two of our midwives were on the way over we knew it meant nothing in terms of when this baby would begin to emerge. So, we never allowed ourselves to anticipate anything specifically. In the thirty minutes or so that it took our midwives to arrive, my contractions progressed from making me lightly moan through them to me writhing in "pain" (I hesitate to use this word, as it feels nothing like the typical pain that we feel). It is different. Labor pains signify progress. It is not such an empty and desperate feeling as is the pain of spraining an ankle. Keep in mind that we never got to set up the birthing tub. Our midwives arrived at 5:15 AM. They set up the bed and an oxygen tank, just in case there were any problems. An herbal compresses was made for my swollen parts during and after the labor. Soups and juices were also prepared for me. Eric's support, herbal compresses, and the caresses of Eric and the midwives were incredible. It was quiet, dark, and beautiful. There were no lights. The only sounds were my moaning, breathing, and a short period of downright screaming. Oh yeah, and the occasional jokes that I made in between contractions. This created a light laughter from the mouths of the three present. You have to keep it light. I was hurting physically, but I felt so good and empowered. It was a very spiritual moment.

Very soon after, I suddenly felt like I needed to push. I was a little shocked by the feeling since I had mentally prepared myself not to feel that feeling for a full day, so I asked my midwives if what I was feeling was okay. They said, "If you feel like you need to push, then push!" Elijah was out at 7:57AM. The room was so warm and cozy. The only light present came from the corners of the shades. All was pleasantly calm and quiet. I stared at him in shock. I processed the fact that we were meeting eye to eye for the first time. After twenty-three minutes he found my breast with no guidance. I was once again reassured by the power of nature and instinct. It is all there; we've just forgotten it because our culture doesn't support it.

As I read over what I've written, I realize that it sounds unnaturally calm. Well, ironically enough this calm is what is natural. The frenzy that we usually hear of is more unnatural than ever. The process-our-process was truly as calm as I've written. It was beautiful. It was incredible. It was empowering for all involved, and it will continue to be.

We had an amazing amount of support for the following six weeks postpartum. Elijah and I never left our room for the first five days. Food and drink were brought to me. We kept the heat up high so that neither of us needed to be clothed, allowing us to be skin - on -skin. On the fifth day, we ventured out into the living room with the curtains drawn. Sometime in the second week of Elijah's life we took a slow walk around the block. I wore him in a wrap on my body. He was asleep and his face was covered, shielding him from the harsh light that he had yet to experience. After two weeks we emerged, but only had outings every now and again. We re-entered the world very slowly and peacefully, knowing that the world would be there waiting for us; but the level of peace that we were experiencing would only last for as long as we allowed it to.

A friend came and stayed with us for two weeks, beginning on Elijah's fifth day of life. She supported us by providing yummy, healthy foods, and just plain old lending us some beautiful female energy. She left us with a freezer full of food which we added to all of the other homemade healthy food provided to us. I didn't have to cook a meal for a full six weeks.

Life has been blissful and peaceful for us as a family. I credit this to the foresight we had as parents-to-be and the research we did. We made peaceful choices and continue to make them. We had warm support from family, friends, and midwives. We worked hard to maintain positive attitudes. I feel blessed that we've been able to do things as we have. I recognize that not all people have this choice, especially in western culture. It is not cheap and it is not readily available. In other places, this is the way it happens. Moms and babies don't leave their homes for weeks, food is provided, and female energy bursts within their walls. It is healthy and peaceful. It is natural. Some people call natural "primitive" with distaste. We have lost that. My wish is that we, as a culture, regain it.

Cris Nicole is the thirty-two-year-old mother of seven-month-old Elijah Kahlil. This involved mother once thought she would never want to parent a child. The thought of being pregnant horrified her. But, here she is, having birthed naturally in her home, breastfeeding, making her own baby food, and using cloth diapers. She has gone as far as to quit her job as a social worker so that she would be able to raise her child in the way that she believes it should be done. Cris has figured out a way to contribute to the household financially while being able to practice natural and attachment parenting to the fullest. No life decision has ever made her more content.

The Birth of Kumara Femi, the Birth of Me
By Aremisa Haile

December 2005
I felt the flutter of little feet hit the walls of my belly. It was true, after months of agonizing over the possibility of being pregnant, at that moment it was confirmed. Sure, my woman's intuition told me that I was with child, but I could not fathom the thought. I had just given birth that past June to a beautiful baby girl, not to

mention we were blessed out of an unfortunate situation to have my wonderful step-son with us full-time. In such a short amount of time I went from care free me, to wife, and soon again mother to be. Now I had to think and I had to think quick, because I was speculated to be 5 ½ months pregnant. How was I going to divide my attention, love, and time between a four-year-old, a toddler, and a newborn baby? I worked in the public school system before with hundreds of kids calling me Mama T, but at the end of the day it was just me. I knew I had to call on my inner strength, but I had to find it first.

April 2006
The overall pregnancy was exhausting and emotional. By, the beginning of April I still did not have a name for this beautiful surprise. My daughter Nekaybaw was crawling and getting into everything and my son Afu-Ra (who was very comfortable calling me mom now) had a never ending supply of questions. My husband and I had just started getting our business off the ground and we had become very active in our Afrikan study group. Things were good and there was a sense of stability. Still deep down I could not shake the fear of keeping it all together when the new baby arrived. One thing was certain; I had to carry my baby to full-term. Although, with Nekaybaw I was seeing my midwife; complications forced us into a hospital birth at twenty-nine weeks of pregnancy. My little warrior princess spent five long weeks in the ICU. Things had to be different. I could not allow my fears to put me in that position again. I began calling out to Yemaya, Osun, and all of the mothers before me to assist with the healthy development of this child. I think I had found my inner strength. I felt renewed. I began to ask my unborn child what lesson she had for me.

May 2006
On the eve of my daughter's arrival I lay in the bed of the birthing center trying to make a compromise with my body as the contractions grew stronger. My midwife was calmly making sure everything was in order, while my husband Malikk, a certified Reiki master, laid his warm hands across my womb and my back. The heat felt so good and seemed to calm me down. I only wanted myself and Malikk in the room. I knew from previous experience

that the energy of friends and family could be a bit overwhelming. It was now 2:30 in the morning and I had been going back and forth from the Jacuzzi tub to the bed as the contractions hovered over my entire body. I was fully dilated, but my bag still had not broken. My midwife, Dinah went in and successfully broke the bag. Then whoosh, all the fears and emotion that I had experienced came out with that last contraction and were replaced by some super power strength. This was definitely different. Although, I had given birth less than a year before, Nekaybaw was three pounds and I was mounted in one position with a nurse holding my legs. I was covered up and unable to see my daughter coming out. This birth was something else. I was bare-naked and very uninhibited physically. I realized my mind had to be as well in order to have a successful birthing experience. I moved around a bit until I found a position that was comfortable. I first was on my knees, then my side, and finally on my back. Now it was time. I pushed, pushed, and pushed. A few times I felt like I wanted to give up. I could feel the presence of my ancestors and all the mothers before me in that room, especially my grandmother Lullaby. In my head I was calling on them for some more strength. I was tired, but determined. Then the head began to peak through. Malikk was holding my hand telling me I was almost there. Dinah offered me a mirror, but I refused. I was too focused. I needed to keep it going. Suddenly, it felt like a small boulder had pushed its way through my legs. The head was out. A few more pushes and out came the shoulders, then the rest of her little body. Kumara Femi was born and so was I. Dinah laid her naked body on my chest and all I saw was a beautiful dimple in her left cheek. She has been here before, I thought. From that moment on I knew that I had the power to turn any negative thought or emotion into something positive, a force to be reckoned with. I realized that I was using my fear and anxiety to control a situation that was governed by Universal Truth. The real control came when I was mentally free and uninhibited, just like giving birth naturally. The real control came when I was in accordance with what the Universe had planned for me. There are no mistakes, just the ones we make by going against what is to be. I use these pearls of wisdom in everything that I do. I have learned to call on the Great Mothers for guidance. The fear and anxiety are gone and I am whole. I now can lead my family to the Promise Land. Thank you Kumara Femi for the lesson.

Aremisa Haile, medicine woman and healer, lives in Dallas,Texas with her husband Malikk and children, Afu-Ra, Nekaybaw, and Kumara. Together they own and operate Indigenous Remedies, a resource for herbal and holistic sciences. For more information their website is www.indigenousremedies.com.

RAHJA AMEN-SUNDJATA
By Roz Fattaleh

Our beautiful baby boy was born April 29th, 2006 at 3:35 A.M., via a beautiful water birth. Rahja Amen-Sundjata was delivered by my amazing husband, wow what a man!! He was perfect. Rahja was 8 lbs 9oz and 20 1/2 inches long. My labor was five hours and hurt something serious. But, with my king by my side and serious meditation, including hypnobirthing, I did it all natural without medication. This was a major difference from my last child, who only weighed five pounds and was seventeen inches. My labor with him was natural as well and lasted the same amount of time. However, the pain was mild compared to this birth. I strongly promote hypnobirthing to all my sistas that are striving to have a natural birth. I learned that birthing does not have to be scary or full of tension, but a natural process. When we take control of our mind and bodies we can alleviate the pain. This allows our babies to come into the world peacefully and smoothly. It is some what like yoga breathing; you are breathing your baby down through the surges (contractions). You are breathing into the pressure instead of fighting or tensing up. I am a pretty high fire individual and sometimes it is hard for me to relax, but with deep breathing and focus I did it with ease.

We were truly blessed to have one more child. We gave thanks for all the blessings and well wishes. Our sunz name is Rahja (Sanskrit for king) Amen (Khemetic for the hidden GOD) Sundjata (the benevolent). Sundjata was the great king of Mali, also spelled Sundiata!! We love him. I must say to all my sistas that if you can have a water birth, do it!! It was a truly uplifting and relaxing experience. I had planned on having one with

Serigne, my oldest son. But, he was a month early. My midwife was concerned about his lungs and vital organs not being fully prepared. So, I just had a natural labor, but looking back I could of had him in water easily. I had done much research on water birthing before I ever had children. I knew that our connection to water as women and child bearers was a perfect entry for my baby. I had read and understood while in the womb a baby is more connected to psychic and spiritual energies. Water being a conductor of energy would help maintain that connection. I believe that the transition for a baby from water to water is a lot less stressful on their little bodies then coming into the world in a hospital full of bright lights with nurses and doctors pulling and tugging at them to come out the womb. Babies are natural swimmers and what better place for their first swimming lesson than the birthing experience. And for the mothers, the feeling of weightlessness is amazing; no hospital bed can make me feel that relaxed. I was able to focus only on my body and my baby.

Before I got into the tub I was in a lot of pain. Once I was submerged in water so much pressure was taken of my body. I could float, turn, and move with such ease. Every time I would feel a surge I could breathe into it instead of trying to get comfortable on a bed, having all my body weight holding me down. Finally, Rahja came so smoothly and peacefully. He did not even cry. He was one with the water, as if he never left the womb. I allowed him to float there and relax for a while instead of having him pulled away from me, cleaned, and weighed, all of that routine hospital crap they put mothers and babies through. Not to mention he got his first bath at the same time he was born, without disturbing him. We let him float until the umbilical cord stopped pulsating. My husband then cut it, by then Rahja was so relaxed he came out the water with ease and began to nurse with no problems. Sistas take control of your bodies and childbirth, consider water birth.

I give thanks to the creator for such an amazing baby, husband, and my other children who are my heart, and can't get enough of their baby brother. This prince like all the newborns coming into this world will lead us into the future and bring us back to our rightful place!! Do it natural sistas and brothas. Promote natural childbirth and breastfeeding.

YOU ARE MY SON
YOU ARE MY SON
YOU ARE MY SUNSHINE
SHINE FOR THE WORLD TO SEE

I FOUND OUT YOU WERE COMING TO THIS WORLD
THEN WONDERED IF YOU WERE A BOY OR GIRL
STARTED TO WORRY ABOUT ALL YOUR NEEDS
REMEMBERED JAH PROVIDES FOR ALL HER SEEDS

DA MONTHS GO BY YOU AND MY BELLY GROW
DEY TELL US YOU'RE A BOY SO NOW WE KNOW
WE DECIDE TO HAVE YOU BORN AT HOME
CUZ HOSPITALS WE CHOOSE TO LEAVE ALONE

DELIVERED SAFELY BY MIDWIFE AND DAD
I HEAR U CRY AND IT MAKES ME SO GLAD
WHEN MORNING COMES U RISE AND MAKE ME SMILE
FOR YOU I'D CRAWL EVEN A THOUSAND MILES

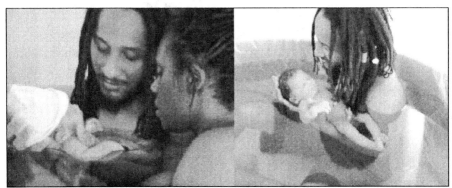

Courtesy of Dera, Photography by Rolanda Robinson

Dera and Emmanuel

57

4 - Postpartum

The Placenta

Placenta burial is a blessing for the child, mother, and earth. In many Afrikan societies placenta burial is considered a rite of passage. Placentas are not simply discarded like pieces of trash. The child's placenta is not to be used in cosmetics or laboratories. It has a spiritual significance and connection to the child. The placenta was a nourishing life force for the baby in the womb. It too was the child's mother. As Afrikans we honor all that is divine and sacred. Placenta burial also promotes womb healing for the mother. The earth too receives nourishment from the placenta. This ceremony is a whole ritual, it is holistic. Parents who choose hospital births may have a hard time taking the placenta home; hospitals have regulations. The placenta can be preserved in the freezer until the ritual is ready to be performed. Family, friends, and elders come to the ceremony. It is usually buried in the family yard or a designated field. The placenta should be thanked for protecting the child during the nine month journey. Libation, prayers, and affirmations can be done. The ritual can be performed in ways to fit each family's lifestyle. The ceremony can be followed with song, dance, and a feast. Make it a blessed event.

In Burkina Faso, West Africa a hole is dug in the ground, and a clay pot with the placenta is placed there. A tree is then planted on top of the pot in such a way that it still receives nutrients from the tree. This spot becomes a place where the child goes to reconnect with his or her source, roots, and origins.[1] The Ibo people of Nigeria and Ghana are said to treat the placenta as the baby's dead twin, and to give it full burial rites.[2]

I buried my son's placenta when he was nineteen-months-old. I held on to his placenta for an unusually long time. I think the placenta was a source of comfort for me and my son. I saw nothing unusual about having a placenta in my freezer. Eventually, I realized that the placenta had done its work and it was time to let go. The ceremony was held in my mother's back yard because my back yard is cement only. My son slept through the ritual. When he woke up he was very irritated. He cried most of the day and into the night. It seemed as though he was not ready to let go of his other mother. I had heard of the strong spiritual bond between placenta and baby. On this day I was actually able to experience it. I was able to fully understand the sacredness of the placenta. I often wonder how my son's emotional and spiritual well being would have been affected if the placenta did not receive proper burial.

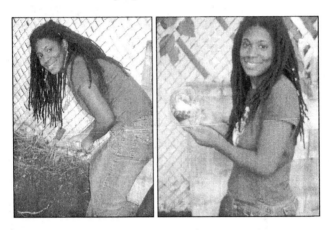

Time of Rest
Once a mother gives birth in many Afrikan countries she is taken care of by the community. She is usually relieved of her normal household duties. Bantu mothers have an n'sansi (nurse girl). She lives with the mother for a few months. She helps the mother with her duties. In Somalia, after a woman gives birth, the family members take care of the mother for forty days. She is to do no housework, she simply cleans herself and breastfeeds the baby. The mother is not obligated to soothe the child either. All the child-holding and bathing and everything is done by her relatives or even by her neighbors.[3] This forty day period is called afatanbah. During this period special meals and teas are prepared for the mother. Mother and baby wear amulets to ward off negative energy. Forty days a celebration takes place followed by a naming ceremony. It is very similar for Ghanaian mothers. She too only has to take good care of herself and nurses the baby. She does not leave the home for 40 days; the family will take care of

59

her. The mother has a special diet. Her intake of sugary foods is restricted for fear of postpartum hemorrhage and for fear that the baby will develop colic and diarrhea. She is given highly nourishing meals which contain herbs that are thought to expel blood clots in the uterus and to promote lactation.[4] After the 40 day period a celebration takes place for the mother of child. This period is seen as the time where the danger is over. A special ceremony is then held for the mother and child; they are dressed well and their bodies are decorated with white clay. Traditional dishes are prepared for friends, relatives, husband, and family.[4] In the United States most mothers do not have a forty day rest. Some mothers are even forced to go to work within thirty days. Many mothers in the United States also experience postpartum depression. The fact that they do not have continuous family support for the first forty days could be a factor. Afrikan communities in the Diaspora must take heed. A network must be established for women so their babies too can reach their full potential. In 1956 Marcelle Geber went to Afrika to study the effects of malnutrition in infants and development. In Uganda she found the infants were more advanced than Western children. These infants were awake a surprising amount of the times - alert, watchful, happy, and calm. They virtually never cried. The mother responded to the infant's every gesture and assisted the child in any and every move that was under taken so that every move initiated by the child ended in immediate success.[5] The Ugandan babies sat upright at two days of birth and were crawling at six or seven weeks.

Circumcision
Many Afrikan parents in the Diaspora have their sons circumcised in the hospitals. Circumcision is pretty much routine. In some cases this procedure is chosen by the parents because they are of a particular religion or culture. Most Afrikans in the United States choose circumcision because they have simply been conditioned to do so. It is not something many parents think of questioning. Some parents believe circumcision promotes cleanliness and decreases the transfer of sexually transmitted diseases. These ideas however are untrue. Many Afrikan parents are unaware of the history of circumcision and the Afrikan man. Afrikan males were targeted more than their White counterparts due to racism.

The incidence of the operation also varies within racial groups. Schrek and Lenowitz demonstrated that early circumcision is more frequently performed in Negroes than in white men.[6] It was believed Afrikans were over sexed and more prone to sexually transmitted diseases. These are obviously racial stereotypes that are not based on research. Oddly, many people today believe there is a link between STDS and the foreskin. The American Academy of Pediatrics found there are not enough benefits of circumcision to advocate the practice for all newborn infants.

Today, the circumcision rate in the United States has dropped to below 60 percent-and as low as 34 percent in Western states, according to the National Center for Health Statistics of the United States Department of Health and Human Services.[7] Circumcision will not decrease urinary tract infections, STDs, or penile cancers. An uncircumcised penis is clean and should not be considered as bad hygiene. As stated earlier the Afrikan man was especially targeted for circumcision. Western society has always had an obsession with the Afrikan penis. Superstitions and myths were created about the size of the Afrikan man's penis and his sex drive. Even today he is blamed for the spread of sexually transmitted diseases. White men believed and still believe he has to protect the White woman from this diseased and over sexed Black buck. Dr. Eugene Hand wrote about the "promiscuous" Afrikan male:

> Circumcision is not common among Negroes. When done it often is later in life and frequently is due to recurrent venereal disease. The sex education of most Negroes is meager. They tend to accept venereal disease with less fear or social taboo than do most Jews and gentiles. Many Negroes are promiscuous. In Negroes there is little circumcision, little knowledge or fear of venereal disease and promiscuity in almost a hornet's nest of infection. Thus the venereal rate in Negroes has remained high.[8]

In the late 1800s, Dr. Peter Charles Remondino was one of the vocal advocates of circumcision. Doctors such as him wanted to enforce the circumcision of all Afrikan males to protect white women from rape. He believed circumcision would also be a means of keeping the Negro clean because he was too ignorant to understand hygiene. Remondino wanted to make it a law that all

61

Afrikan males be circumcised.   *The Maryland Medical Journal* agreed with Remondino stating:

> He has observed that whilst male Jews are noted for their strong sexual proclivities, such a character as a Jewish rapist is never heard of. He attributes this fact to the practice of circumcision, and he now suggests that the legal enforcement of circumcision among the Negro race would effectually remedy the predisposition to aping inherent in this race.[9]

Many might wonder how the medical industry convinced parents to get their children circumcised regardless of their religious or cultural beliefs. Dr. David Chamberlin explains:

> Circumcision originated at least 6,000 years ago as a tribal and religious identity symbol in Semitic cultures. The ballooning of the practice in 20th century America was the work of pediatricians and obstetricians who gave it new status as a "medical" procedure. Circumcision also received a big lift from a wealthy layman, John Harvey Kellogg, founder of the cereal company, who was obsessed with the evils of masturbation and advocated circumcision as the solution. Kellogg's book, *Plain Facts for Old and Young,* urged parents to have their boys circumcised without anesthesia--because the pain would have a "salutory effect upon the mind"--and was as common in American homes at the time as his corn flakes.[10]

Breastfeeding

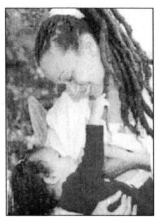

*Courtesy of Venus Paloma Rodriguez-McGregor,
Photography by Dyana Van Campen*

Breastfeeding is one of the greatest gifts a woman can give her child. It is the perfect food for baby because breast milk is specially designed for the baby. Breastfeeding helps to prevent allergies, asthma, ear infections, meningitis, obesity, cancer, hospitalization, and much more. Breastfed babies are also smarter than non–breastfed babies and have increased cognitive development. Here are some breastfeeding benefits:

- Breastfeeding promotes womb healing. The uterus is allowed to naturally contract and reduce hemorrhaging.
- Breastfeeding burns calories, allowing the body to get back in shape faster.
- Exclusive breastfeeding delays ovulation for most women during the first six months and acts as a natural contraceptive method. However, every woman's body is different.
- Breastfeeding helps to prevent breast and ovarian cancer.
- Breastfeeding can prevent postpartum depression. Oxytocin is secreted during breastfeeding creating feelings of joy and love. Breastfeeding mothers are happier moms.
- Breastfeeding can help to prevent osteoporosis.

Breastfeeding also benefits the environment. The earth which sustains the Afrikan family must be protected. Mothers especially must do their part to protect the mother called earth. The Pan – African magazine *Black Woman and Child* states:

> Infant formulas are recalled on a regular basis because of industrial and bacterial contamination. On top of all that, fossil fuels, wood, and other kinds of resources are used up. Forests are cut down to make room for cows to graze to make the milk on which formulas are based. The production of wastes, including green house gasses, manufacturing and use of metals, plastics, and paper for packaging are all a big part of the formula production industry.[11]

So, why are so many women using formula? In 1867, Henri Nestlé put a mixture of flour and condensed milk onto the market. In 1872 his business sold five million cartons of this "formula" around the world.[11] Today billions of dollars are made each year by the formula industry. The campaigns used are very aggressive. Formula is marketed as being like breast milk. Parents are given free breast milk samples before leaving the hospital. When you add the media and society's negative opinions about breastfeeding, formula becomes the ideal choice for some mothers.

Breastfeeding provides more than just nutritional health benefits. Mothers pass on their love, history, and essence. The child no longer lives in the womb and the umbilical cord is cut. But the mother still has the physical and spiritual tie of the breast. The Dogon of Mali have a proverb, "The breast is second only to god." Babies are receiving not only nourishment, but divine nourishment. The placenta sustained the baby's life, now the breast is a life giver. Some women do not breastfeed because they think there is something sexual about the act. In many Afrikan tribes women freely walk around bare breasted. The breasts are not taboo or looked at as sexual objects. The Afrikan woman in America has been affected by Eurocentric perversions. Breasts are a symbol of fertility and womanhood. They are the connection to the Ra, the life force. Afrikans have let today's society dictate who the creator is. The Afrikan woman is the creator. Her breast gave life to Afrika. Mothers can give their babies Afrika through their breast milk. Nursing mothers must not only eat well, just as they did when pregnant, but also feed their mental being with healthy foods. Emotions and thoughts are also passed through breast milk. Peaceful foods and thoughts must be consumed. The breast must be loved and honored. Oil and massage them daily. Keep them healthy for the baby. If salves or oils are used, make sure these are not harmful to the baby.

It is important mothers breastfeed their newborns as soon as possible after birth. The longer they wait, the harder it is for the baby to latch on. The more natural the birth with minimal medicalization, the easier breastfeeding is for mother and baby. Pacifiers and bottles must be avoided for mothers who plan to breastfeed. Even if the milk takes 3-5 five days to come in, avoid bottles. The colostrum present in the breast after the birth is sufficient and full of nutrients. Colostrum also provides antibodies to protect the baby from illness.

Some mothers experience pain while breastfeeding. If the baby's latch is painful, the mouth may not be open wide over the areola. The baby's lips are not supposed to be only latched onto the nipple. Mothers with severe issues breastfeeding should contact a lactation consultant, doula, or even a sista friend before giving up. Many pediatricians are not knowledgeable about breastfeeding, consult a lactation consultant first. Nursing mothers do not nurse on a schedule like those bottle feeding. Nursing is done on demand. This supplies the baby with the nutrients needed and keeps the mother's milk supply up.

Returning to work does not have to deter mothers from breastfeeding. While the mother is at home she can nurse her baby on one side and pump on the other. The pumped milk is then stored in the freezer. The best pumps for mothers pumping half-time are the double electric pumps. I used the Medela Pump In Style©. It is great for mothers who are pumping regularly such as during the day, while at work. Many mothers feel their employers will not let them pump at work. Mothers in the workplace have rights. Before returning to work or accepting a new job, mothers can explain to their employers they will be nursing their child. Many employers will set up a lactation room or allow mothers to use a vacant office. If all else fails she may have to pump in the bathroom or in the car. Mothers should breastfeed their babies before leaving for work in the morning. Baby - sitters or daycare providers should be advised to hold off on feeding the baby close to the time the mother will arrive for pick up. This allows the baby to breastfeed upon the mother returning. Bottles should be avoided for morning, night, and weekend feedings. This will keep the milk supply up.

Storing Breast Milk
Pumped milk that cannot be immediately refrigerated is safe to leave out for 6-8 hours. Breast milk keeps in the refrigerator for eight days. It can remain in the freezer for 3-6 months. Deep freezers enable milk to keep for up to a year. Only freeze milk in a container approved for storing breast milk in the freezer. Use freezer bags (not sandwich bags) or breast milk storage bags. Thaw breast milk in the refrigerator. Never microwave breast milk. Simply run it under hot water or place in a hot cup of water when preparing to warm for baby. Do not re-freeze thawed milk. Breast milk can be re-used for another feeding. Parents do not have to throw away unfinished breast milk.

Some moms experience low milk supply. This is not a reason to throw in the towel. Herbs called galactagogues are frequently used, they increase milk supply. Galactagogues such as fenugreek, blessed thistle, and alfalfa can be used. They can be taken as a tea, tincture or capsule. Most mothers take fenugreek in capsule form. I sometimes would make a tea consisting of fenugreek, alfalfa, and red raspberry. Red Raspberry makes the breast milk high in nutrients. Nettle and oat straw are also great herbs to help enhance breast milk.

Baby Food
The baby's first food should be breast milk. Some mothers feed their children solids sometime after five-months-of-age. Others wait until one-years-of-age. There is no reason to give children before five months of age cereal or any other type of solid. Many grandmothers and great-grandmothers will encourage mothers to feed their babies solids as young as one month. Babies cannot digest foods properly this early. Breast milk is all the child needs. Breastfeeding mothers run the risk of decreasing their milk supply

if solids are started too soon. The baby will spend less time on the breast and more time eating solids. Breastfeeding is about supply and demand. Mothers who cannot breastfeed due to health reasons or other factors should use formula only before five-months-of-age. Parents should not begin solids just because their child has reached the five month mark. They should wait until the child is ready.

- The baby should know how to sit upright, having head control.
- The baby should have an appetite for solids. If the baby is still hungry after eight or more feedings, solids may be an option.
- The baby should attempt chewing motions. The tongue should move food back, not forward. If the tongue pushes forward the baby is not ready for solids.

Introducing Solids
Continue to breastfeed on demand. If baby is drinking expressed milk during the day, the bottles provided should not be decreased before eight-months-of-age. Breast milk should be the baby's primary food source even when starting solids. The baby should be breastfeeding at least five times a day or drinking 32 ounces of formula a day. If the baby is not drinking this amount, decrease the amount of solid foods.[12] The first and last meal of the day should always be breast milk. A little water in a sippy cup can be provided for in between meals. Parents should begin with one meal per day. Some breast milk should be given first, followed by solids, water, and then the remaining breast milk. Parents can move towards two meals a day when the baby is ready.

Many babies have rice cereal as their first food. They usually do not have allergic reactions to rice. Organic whole grain cereals can be purchased from health food stores or markets. Parents can also make their own cereals. But be mindful that home-made cereals are not iron fortified. Whole grain cereals can be made by grinding organic oats, millet, or brown rice in a blender or grinder. Use ¼ cup of the grain, 1 cup of water, and cook. Home - made cereals are not recommended for children under six months.

Making your own baby foods are best, followed by commercial organic baby foods. When making baby foods use clean hands and utensils. Wash all fruits and vegetables thoroughly. Use organic foods whenever possible. To make your own baby foods simply steam your vegetables and fruits and puree in a blender. Boiling foods causes loss of nutrients. Parents batch cooking foods can store small amounts of foods in the freezer, using freezer bags. Food can also be frozen in ice cube trays and placed in bags. The appropriate cube amount needed can be taken out of the freezer bag for each feeding. Cubes are ideal because they are small serving sizes. Freezer bags can be expensive. Small portions of food can be stored in cheaper sandwich bags and then placed in one big freezer bag. Label your freezer bags with dates. Freezable jars are available, if you can find them. If you cannot find them you can re-use freezer bags to save money and the environment. Simply wash the freezer bags and use them again. Do not keep frozen baby food over two months. Place food to be thawed in the refrigerator the night before. Do not use microwaves. Microwaves emit radiation, which cause cancer. Food that has been thawed should not be frozen again. Discard of refrigerated foods after two days. New foods should be introduced every seven days. So, if an allergic reaction occurs the parent will know what food caused it. Fruits should be peeled. Pits and seeds should be removed. Sugars and salts should not be added to baby foods. Feed children the appropriate food for their age. Do not give children less than one-year-of-age strawberries, citrus fruits, honey, or cow's milk.

Some Suggested Foods

6 mths	7 mths	8 mths	9 mths	10 -12 mths
cereal avocado banana sweet potatoes plums peaches apricots pears green beans *cook all fruits, except bananas and avocados until 7 months of age*	squash peas carrots Mango papaya diluted fruit juice	apples waterm elon broccol i cauliflo wer kiwi	green leafy vegetables (spinach, collards, kale, etc.) beans(wit hout skin)	whole grain pasta

When the child becomes a toddler try combinations such as steamed vegetables with rice, millet, couscous, quinoa, yams, cassava, or sweet potatoes. Pastas and stews are also great toddler foods.

Cloth Diapering

Cloth diapering is a healthy and economical choice for families. It is also healthy for the earth. There are so many reasons to cloth diaper. Most disposable diapers have chemicals and are bleached with chlorine. The chlorine creates dioxin, which is toxic. The effects of polyacrylate gel in the diapers, used to keep the diaper dry, are unknown. Children's skin is sensitive along with their immune systems. Surround children with a natural and holistic environment. Not only is the child's immediate environment important, but so is the global environment. Disposable diapers are harmful to the ecosystem. Compared to cloth diapers throw away diapers use 20 times more raw materials, three times more energy, and twice as much water; they generate 60 times more waste.[13] Afrikans understand God is connected to the earth. It is against the laws of Maat to pollute the earth. Cloth diapering is also better for children's health. A study in the September 1999 issue of *Archives of Environmental Health* found that laboratory mice exposed to various brands of throwaway diapers suffered eye, nose, and throat irritation, including bronchoconstriction similar to that resulting from an asthma attack.[13] Another great reason to use cloth over disposable diapers is the economic benefit. The most money I spent on diapers for my son's first year of life was $150.00. Thousands of dollars can be spent depending on how long the child is in diapers. Cloth diapering also helps with early potty training.

Cloth diapers now come in many varieties. No longer do parents have to use pins and plastic pants. Nor, is the folding complicated. Parents can choose from a multitude of fabrics including organic cotton, hemp, fleece, wool, velour , and more. These cloth diapers cannot be found in most stores. They are sold online, usually by WAHMS (Work At Home Moms).

Types of Cloth Diapers
Prefolds – A prefolded piece of cloth. Indian and Chinese cotton prefolds diapers are most popular. They are also available in hemp and fleece. A cover is used to hold the prefold in place. One of the best advantages of prefolds is the price. They can be brought for as low as $1.00 each.
Fitted – Fitted diapers come in many sizes. They require no folding, they are fitted. They come with buttons, snaps, or velcro. They look like disposable diapers, only cloth. A cover must be purchased. Diapers range between $8.00-$15.00.
Pocket – Pocketed diapers look like fitted diapers, but need no cover. Inserts are added in the pocket for absorbency. They usually have a fleece lining. Diapers range between $10.00-$16.00.
All In Ones – All In Ones are fitted and there is no need for a cover or pocket insert. Diapers range between $15.00-$25.00.

Diaper Covers – Diaper covers are needed for prefolds and fitted diapers only. Covers come in wool, fleece, polyurethane, cotton, and polyester. Diaper covers range between $6.00-$15.00.

Cloth diapering Essentials:
It might be best for moms new to cloth to start out simple when choosing to buy cloth.

Below is what I suggest:

- At least twenty-five prefolds.
- Five diaper covers are recommended. Buy at least one night time cover.
- Two fitted Diapers.
- All In Ones and pocketed diapers are optional. Parents can choose for themselves how many they need. Buy only one or two first, see if they are actually worth it.
- Six fleece liners, the liners keep the baby dry especially over night.

Washing Cloth
Diaper services are available. However, if parents would like to save money they can buy and wash their diapers themselves. When prefold diapers are first purchased they have oils and waxes on them. Wash the diapers first, to guarantee absorbency. Wash prefolds in hot water with detergent at least three times. Diapers must also be dried three times. Pour a few drops of water on the diaper to see if it is absorbent, if the water beads wash them again. Boiling hot water and placing the prefolds in the water for about five minutes instead of washing three times is another option. Be extremely careful when doing this. Tongs can be used.

Washing Routine

- Short wash or pre-rinse prefolds in cold water with a half cup of baking soda. Adding three drops of tea tree oil is optional. The rinse or short wash will depend on whether parents have a top or front loading washer.

- Run a full wash with hot water using natural detergent, using the extra rinse setting. Many parents use Bi-O-Kleen or Allen's Naturally. They are natural and have great stain fighting abilities. The downside of using Bio-Kleen is that its live enzymes can build up and irritate baby's skin. If this happens simply strip the diapers.
- Some families prefer to run another wash with hot water without detergent.

Cloth is usually washed every 2-3 days. Soiled cloth is stored in a dry bucket. Using a dry bucket with no water equals less mess. The use of fabric softener is not recommended. It makes the diapers less absorbent. Many people use a ½ cup of vinegar occasionally to soften diapers. Cloth diapers sometimes experience a build up of detergent, fabric softener, and residue. This can cause the diapers to be less absorbent, smelly, and irritate the baby's skin. The diapers can be stripped to resolve these issues. Stripping is the process of washing them with hot water only until the suds are no longer seen. If you wash them three times, dry them three times.

Diapering is uncommon in many parts of Afrika. In Somalia, when the baby is awake, the mother will hold a small basin in her lap and then hold her baby in a sitting position over the basin at regular time intervals. Somali mothers claim that within a short period of time infants are trained to use the "potty". At nighttime, a piece of plastic is placed between the mattress and the bedding. The bedding and plastic are cleaned daily.[14] While visiting a Ethiopian friend's restaurant; a waitress told me her brother had never worn a diaper. His baby-sitter would sit him on her lap and roll her skirt up. She would open her legs when it was time for him to eliminate. The waste went into a container below. Diasporan Afrikans can ask the Continental Afrikans for advice about infant potty training. There are also books available about early infant potty training, give it a try.

How to use a prefold and wrap

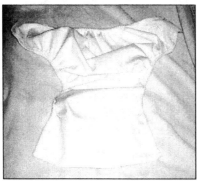

1. Lay the wrap flat.

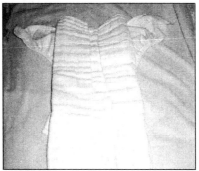

2. Place Chinese prefold on the wrap (Tri-Fold).

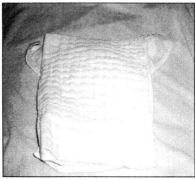

3. Or create a newspaper fold.

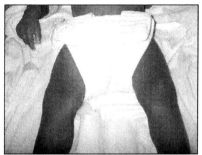

4. Place baby on cloth and position the prefold.

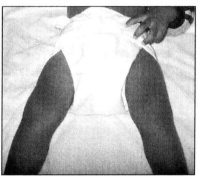

5. Fasten the wrap.

Baby Wearing

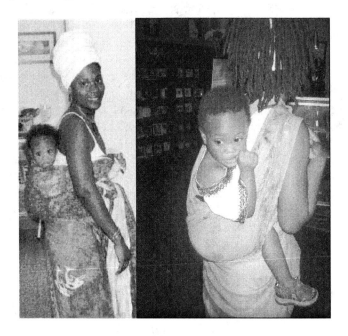

The most beneficial way to transport your baby is to wear your baby, but most Afrikans living in the West use strollers. Jane Clark, professor of kinesiology at the University of Maryland states:

> There was concern that Americans were overusing strollers for older children, causing toddlers to be less physically active. A growing movement among child advocates promotes the idea of carrying babies more and getting them out of their strollers.[15]

Baby wearing has many benefits. It supports bonding, reduces crying, and colic. Baby wearing provides the womb environment the baby is accustomed to. Mother and baby are in synch. The baby is able to hear the mother's heart beat just as she did while in the womb. It creates oneness and security. Baby wearing also is helpful to mothers. It allows her to be hands free while carrying the baby so things such as housework can be done. When the mother is out of the home people passing will be less likely to touch her baby. Baby wearing is also great for potty training.

Most Afrikan mothers on the continent do not use diapers on their babies. They monitor the baby's movements and gestures while wearing them. They then hold the baby over the place chosen for elimination. Across Africa, women can be seen carrying sleeping or sometimes giggly babies on their backs, swathed in cloth. The babies move to the sway of their mother's hips, synchronized throughout the day, bending with them as they collect water or sweep the floor and rising again when the women stop to rest.[15] Baby wearing is also a great tool for daycare providers. Many small babies lay in bassinets most of the time in daycare. Babies need constant touch and love. Daycare providers should consider using slings and/or wraps for the children in their care. Mothers using daycare services can ask their provider if they can use a carrier. The art of baby wearing is essential for the traditional Afrikan baby-sitter. Bringing Afrikan traditional values to the Western daycare system can provide a balance.

There are many options for wearing your babies. The most traditional way is using a simple piece of cloth or sarong. Many options are available if mothers desire other types of carriers. Ring slings, mei tais, wraps, and podaegis are available.

How to Wrap Your Baby with Fabric

Stretchy fabric such as jersey knit can be used to wrap smaller babies. Stronger fabrics such as cotton gauze or knits can be used to wrap larger babies. The wrap can be anywhere from 4 ½-6 inches long. The width can be between 35-45 inches wide. Wraps can be made at home or purchased. Parents who choose to make their own wraps can simply cut the fabric and wear. Or the edges can be sewn or serged. Always make sure your baby is secure, check frequently! Watch out for your baby's limbs and head when walking.

Instructions for a back carry
This carry takes practice. Make sure one hand is always holding the baby. Have someone spot you when learning this carry.

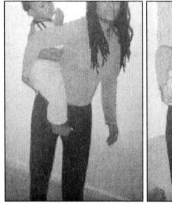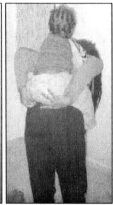

1. Place the baby on your hip, begin to move baby towards your back.
2. Position the baby on your back.

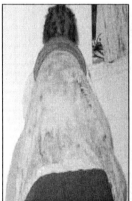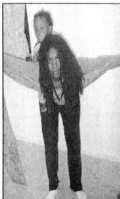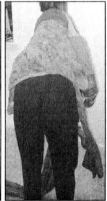

3. Lean forward, drape fabric around the baby.
4. Bring fabric towards your chest and criss-cross.
5. Bring one piece of fabric over your right shoulder. Cross over the baby's back and under the child's left leg. This will also be the left side of your body.

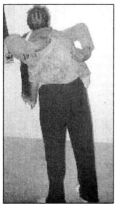 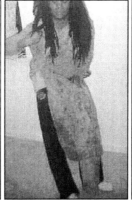 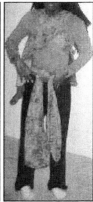

6. Cover the baby's back and place fabric over the baby's bottom and under the leg.
7. Bring fabric from under the baby's leg and bring forward. Repeat steps 6–8 for the opposite side.
8. Bring the remaining fabric to the front and tie. You can make the hold tighter by pulling the pieces tight towards you.

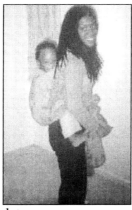 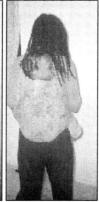

9. Complete

To remove the baby, untie the front knot. Remove the fabric from under each leg and off the baby's back. Hold the baby while doing this. Remove the criss-crossed fabric from your chest while holding the baby firm. Bring baby forward, much like you brought the baby around to your back. While holding the baby, move the baby over to your hips and bring the child to the front of your body.

Instructions for a front carry

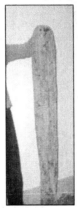

1. Find the center of your cloth.

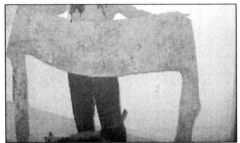

2. Drape cloth across your stomach.

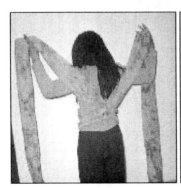 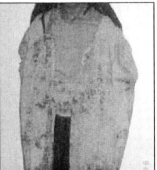

3. Criss–cross both ends across your back.
4. Bring the two end pieces to the front, across your shoulders.

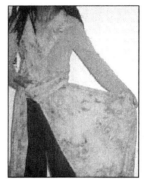

5. Criss-cross the fabric in front of you. Place one end in the belt.

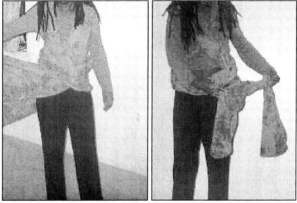

6. Do the same for the opposite end. You will have a cross at your chest. The baby's legs will go here. Make a loose knot at your side.

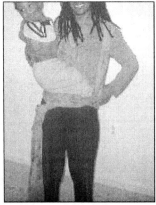

7. Place baby's leg in one side of the cross.

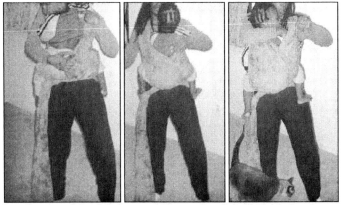

8. Open up the fabric to cover more of the baby's back.
9. Do the same for the opposite leg, steps 7 through 8.
10. Spread fabric across the baby's back for a secure position.

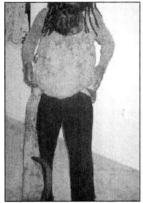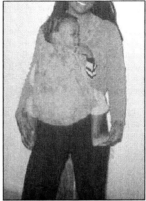

11. Make final adjustments. You can now tighten the knot at your side.
This is also how the fabric should look draped across your baby's back for the back carry.

    12. Complete

For Smaller Babies

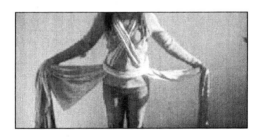

1. Using a stretchy fabric such as jersey knit, repeat Steps 1 through 6 for the previous cross wrap position.

82

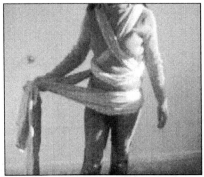

2. There should be extra fabric. Wrap it around your body and make a loose knot at your waist. This will make an extra belt.

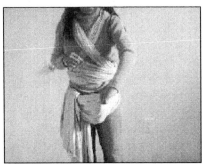

3. Place the baby's legs in the crosses. Pull the top belt over the baby's back. This front cross position provides extra support and security for smaller babies.

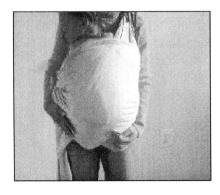

4. Make a knot at your side with the extra belt fabric.

I started babywearing when I had my first son. I would wear him primarily on my back religiously, for the first six months of his life. It was when I tried to put him down that was the problem. He loved being close to the warmth of his mommy and hearing my heartbeat, it soothed him. I wore him until he was about eighteen months. He was a happy baby because of it; the yummy breast milk did not hurt either. My second son also benefited from the comfort and beauty of babywearing. It makes him happy to be so close to me, and to see the world right from my hip or back. I love it and so does he.

Akilah Muhammad
Mommy of two (NYC)

Baby-sitting and Daycare
In today's society a large number of children are in daycare at ages as young as two months. The thought of it is frightening, the large amount of children compared to the small ratio of care givers. My son's baby-sitters are my grandmother, mother, and aunt. His occasional baby-sitter during the weekend is my younger 17-year-old god-sister. I give thanks, honor, and praise to them for making it possible for me to keep my son out of daycare. They have allowed him to have the opportunity to experience an Afrikan holistic way of baby-sitting. In the West, people look at the occupation of baby - sitting to be for the uneducated or for the youth. The people of Kongo call baby-sitting Kindezi, the art of touching, caring for and protecting the child's life and the environment, kinzungidila, in which the child's multidimensional development takes place.[16] Kindezi is considered an art form. Fu-Kiau believes that baby-sitting is a requirement of all members of the Afrikan community. In the West, many mothers work during the day in corporate America or work for themselves. Mothers need someone to mind their children. The Kongo women are farmers. They leave for the fields in the early mornings and come home at night fall. Baby-sitters called ndezis give women the independence to work on the farms, provide resources, and food for their families. Many times ndezis are considered even more mentally healthy than the child's biological parent. This is because the ndezi is directly responsible for the child's well being

and development. There are young and old ndezis. The young
ndezis are between the ages of nine and ten. The ndezi feeds,
bathes, and entertains the child while the mother is away during
the day. Sometimes the ndezi even has food prepared for the
mother when she gets home. The young ndezi is actually being
prepared for motherhood. The old ndezis do not have to work on
farms, so they are perfect. The children keep them busy and deter
loneliness. This also keeps the elder's mind sharp and prevents,
"psychosomatic ailments".[16] The elder ndezis also teach the
younger ndezis. Older ndezis teach the child traditional language,
customs, community life, songs, games, and tricks. They also
educate the children about animals, plants, and reproduction. The
ndezi and child usually learn at sadulu. The sadulu is a simple
baby - sitting site which can be under a tree or in a hut. It is not a
traditional school where you read and write. The teachings are
traditional, oral. Children go out on what people in the West call
field trips. They visit the weavers, farmers, blacksmiths, etc. The
children collect flora, roots, and herbs. They learn about animals
and insects from analyzing and dissecting them. This type of
schooling is frowned upon by the modern Afrikan schools. As a
child I went to Montessori schools. They greatly mimic a sadulu.
Teachings were not traditional. I do not remember a chalkboard,
paper, or pens. I do remember flora, insects, and everyday
household items. There was also a starfish we could analyze. Our
traditional ways have been greatly condemned and at the same
time greatly imitated.

In Afrikan society children are invaluable; they are essential to the
strength of the community. So, they must be honored. An
environment must be created which is whole. The Kongo proverb
says, "The child in the womb is a burden to one person; outside
(born), it belongs to everybody in the community.[16] When my
grandmother was working outside of the home a woman who lived
on the same street watched her children. There was no need for
daycare centers. Today, the elders and young people in the
community are reluctant to become ndezis. This has social and
economic impacts on the communities of the West. The
government is now cutting off welfare for many mothers. So,
mothers must sometime find jobs only paying minimum wage.
These mothers sometimes cannot afford daycare at all or must

choose among the worst daycares. Some mothers cannot afford to work because they must care for their children. Most daycares are not beneficial to the child's development. This is why community is so important. As Afrikans we have to look home to Afrika and seek proper methods for balancing school, work, and parenthood. The Western way is to simply let television baby-sit children. Families are almost forced into situations where complete strangers watch their children. Daycare providers have a great impact on children's development. Children come home today exhibiting behaviors outside of what is allowed in the home. The community needs holistic alternatives. Afrikans must begin sharing and relating with their neighbors and children again. Women must get together and form counsels, addressing the daycare needs in the community. If resources are pooled Afrikans can come up with solutions. It is vital that our communities make use of the people in them again. So, Afrikans can in turn take back their children.

5 - Keeping Your Children Healthy

Vaccinations

A vaccine is a portion of the weakened germ injected into the body. This is supposed to cause the body to produce antibodies against the virus or bacteria, preventing contraction of the actual disease. Vaccinations are credited for the decline of many childhood diseases. However, there is no scientific evidence to prove this. Many of these diseases were on the decline prior to mass vaccination campaigns in the United States. Proper nutrition and sanitation is also an important contribution to the decline. Europe's vaccination campaigns came after the United States'. Yet, Europe still saw a decline. Today, Europe administers fewer immunizations than the United States. In the United States vaccines are a billion dollar business. Vaccines are always being created regardless of whether or not the diseases are fatal or extremely harmful. Worldwide revenues from vaccine development are nearly $3 billion and are expected to more than double to $7 billion over the next five years.[1] Many childhood diseases have declined since mass vaccinations. But other ailments such as allergies, attention deficit disorder, cancer, asthma, speech problems, and mental retardation, and autism have risen. Many physicians can attest to this:

> Michael Odent, MD, and fellow European researchers showed the incidence of asthma is five times greater and of earaches is two times greater in children who have received the whole cell pertussis vaccination than those who have not. Denver physician Philip Incao, MD, reports that 50 percent of the children in his Denver practice are vaccinated, and 50 percent are unvaccinated. He observed that the unvaccinated children usually have an immune system that reacts more responsively and vigorously to acute infections than that of vaccinated children.[1]

Autoimmune disorders have also been on the rise. Autoimmune disorders cause the immune system to attack itself instead of diseases and infections. Foreign DNA in the vaccines which are injected into the body can harm the immune system. Vaccines contain many toxic ingredients including, aborted fetal tissue, formaldehyde, aluminum, ethylene glycol (anti-freeze), phenol, thimerosal (mercury), monkey tissue, pig tissue, rabbit tissue, and chick embryo cells.

Some Afrikan countries have seen an increase of AIDS related symptoms after vaccines have been mass distributed. An immune system can become deficient for a number of reasons, malnutrition, lack of clean water, and toxic chemicals injected into veins, such as vaccines. Afrikans are being labeled with having HIV without even being administered an HIV test. They can receive this label due to diarrhea, coughing, and itchy hands alone. Some Afrikan children are malnourished so when they receive vaccines it takes a huge toll on their bodies, causing AIDS related symptoms. Vaccinations cannot be reversed. All over the world it is quite common for babies to experience fever, irritability, and rashes. Because many children have been injured due to vaccines there is a National Vaccine Injury Program (NVICP), since its inception, the program has received over 500,000 claims for compensation since; 85 percent of these claims were for vaccines administered before 1988. Of those 5,000 claims, over 1,100 awards totaling $800 million in compensation have been made to individuals or familes.[1] *Pediatrics* published a study in which parents were specifically asked to observe any change in their baby's behavior or physical condition after a shot; only seven percent were able to report no reactions at all.[2]

Tetanus
Tetanus is a bacteria found in soil and manure. It usually enters the body through wounds. Tetanus can cause severe muscle spasms, broken bones, and even death. Symptoms may include chills, fever, stiffness of jaw and neck, and irritability. If an unvaccinated child or adult is suspected of having tetanus, a tetanus immune globulin injection can be administered at the time of infection. Many parents are unaware tetanus is unlikely to survive in a shallow wound that bleeds. The disease can only survive and multiply if no oxygen is present. The wound must be kept clean. Deep puncture wounds and wounds with a lot of dead tissue should be thoroughly washed.[2]

Measles

Measles is a contagious viral disease. Measles symptoms include fever, rash, and mucus. Today measles is nearly gone in the United States. However, the vast majority of the cases that do occur are among people who have been immunized.[3] I am one of those people. I had measles as a child. My recovery period consisted of rest at a neighbor's home. My parents had to work during the day. Measles in a healthy child is usually not fatal. Problems can occur in previously sick or malnourished children. The MMR vaccine is one vaccine for all three diseases, mumps, measles, and rubella. Parents can request separate vaccines if they choose to vaccinate. The MMR vaccine has been associated with causing autism. Measles may be resistant to the vaccine, the CDC has identified 8 different genotypes of wild measles virus throughout the world that may have occurred because the vaccine has forced the virus to mutate.[3]

Rubella

Rubella is also viral and contagious. Rubella usually has no symptoms, sometimes there may be a rash. Rubella is harmful to pregnant woman. When rubella occurs during early pregnancy, the result is often congenital rubella syndrome (CRS), which includes miscarriage, stillbirths, fetal anomalies for example, deafness, cataracts, glaucoma, heart defects, mental retardation, bone defects and poor growth) and therapeutic abortions.[3]

Mumps

Mumps is a viral disease. It is associated with fever, swollen salivary glands, and some males experience swollen testicles. In rare cases swelling of the brain and meningitis can occur. The mumps vaccine was actually developed for boys, not girls, to prevent sterilization.

Diphtheria

Diphtheria is a communicable bacterial disease caused by corynebacterium diphtheriae. The greatest number of cases of diphtheria were in 1921 when 206,939 contracted the disease. In 1992, there were only four cases.[1] Symptoms of diphtheria include sore throat, fever, swollen neck lymph nodes, chills, and breathing problems. A membrane forming on the tonsils and throat can cause the breathing difficulties if it extends into the windpipe and lungs. Diphtheria can be treated with penicillin.

Meningitis
Meningitis can be caused by both meningococcal disease and pneumocical disease. Meningococcal Disease is caused by neisseria meningitides, it causes meningitis and meningococcal. Meningococcal causes an infection of the spinal and brain fluid. It also can cause meningococcemia, a blood infection. Pneumococcal disease is caused by the bacteria Streptococcus pneumoniae. Meningitis symptoms include high fever, irritability, restlessness, stiff neck, nausea, and vomiting.

Haemophilus Influenzae Type B (HIB)
Haemophilus Influenzae Type B is a bacterium that lives in the respiratory tract. It is contagious and can be spread through coughing and sneezing. Poor living conditions and compromised immune symptoms increase the risk of infection greatly for children six-years-of-age and under. HIB can cause bacterial meningitis. Symptoms include fever, chills, cough, sleepiness, lack of appetite, stiff neck, vomiting, and convulsions. HIB not treated can cause neurological damage and death.

Chickenpox
Varicella commonly known as chickenpox is a contagious virus. Most children contract the disease and it is usually harmless. Some parents send their children to chickenpox parties so they can catch the disease and simply get it over with. Symptoms include itchy rash and fever. The disease sometimes causes fatal complications in adults who never had chickenpox as a child and sickly children. The chickenpox or varicella vaccine is being pushed not because it is fatal for healthy children, but because it is a nuisance for corporate America. Many parents have to stay home and nurse their children. The vaccine raises a few concerns. Adults who were vaccinated against chickenpox as children may get the virus later in life, when the condition can be more severe. Some parents are concerned that the vaccine contains cells from aborted fetal tissue.

Polio

Polio is an infectious viral illness. Symptoms are similar to the flu and may include diarrhea, fever, cough, and sore throat. However, a small few experience paralysis. Polio is said to be eradicated from the Western Hemisphere. Each year, however, there are five to seven vaccine-related cases of polio in the United States.[1] Some medical professionals believe pollution, arsenic, and pesticides such as DDT have attributed to polio outbreaks of the past. DDT kills flies. It was once believed flies carried the polio virus. DDT is being considered to control the spread of malaria in Afrika. Many polio cases are now diagnosed as meningitis:

> The standards for defining polio were changed when the live-virus polio vaccine was introduced. The new definition of a polio epidemic required more cases to be reported. Paralytic polio was redefined as well, making it more difficult to confirm and tally cases. Prior to the introduction of the vaccine the patient only had to exhibit paralytic symptoms for 24 hours. Laboratory confirmation test to determine residual (prolonged) paralysis were not required. The new definition required the patient to exhibit paralytic symptoms for at least 60 days, and a residual paralysis had to be confirmed twice during the course of the disease. Also, after the vaccine was introduced cases of aseptic meningitis (an infectious disease that is difficult to distinguish from polio) and coxsackie virus infections were reported as separate diseases from polio.[2]

Pertussis

Pertussis, also known as whooping cough is an infectious disease caused by bacteria. Many people call it the three month cough. This cough can last weeks or months. The coughing spells can be very severe. Mucous builds up in the lungs causing violent coughing spells which can cause breathing difficulties. There is no cure pertussis. Many parents and their children have been able to get through whooping cough using sodium acsorbate. Mothers with newborns take it orally, so the baby receives it through breast milk. It also can be placed in bottles. Doctors have found ascorbic acid reduces the intensity of the disease. Some children do require medicalization, but many times antibiotics are not effective. The DPT vaccine is administered to prevent diphtheria, pertussis, and tetanus. Parents commonly report adverse reactions after their children have received the DTP vaccine. Adverse reactions such as irritability, seizures, developmental delays, diarrhea, vomiting, breathing problems, shock, and death have been reported. Recent scientific studies have linked SIDS and breathing difficulties such as apnea, and hypopnea with pertussis vaccinations. A DTaP vaccine was created and marketed as being less toxic.

Hepatitis B
Hepatitis B is a viral disease. The virus attacks the liver and may cause serious damage. It can only be transmitted through bodily fluids, such as those exchanged during sexual intercourse or intravenous drug use. Most hospitals give infants the hepatitis B vaccine not too long after birth. I personally do not know of any infants who use drugs or are sexually active. The hepatitis B vaccine has been linked with multiple sclerosis. A recent study conducted by Dokuz Eylul University's Department of Neurology found:

> The aetiology of multiple sclerosis (MS) is still not fully understood. Infectious agents are believed to play a role in the development of this multifactorial disease. Cases in which this disease occurs after administration of both plasma-derived and recombinant hepatitis B vaccines have been reported. In this study, we compared a group of 11 MS patients who developed first clinical symptoms after hepatitis B vaccination (group I) with 71 MS patients who were never vaccinated against hepatitis B and were negative for hepatitis B serology (group II), and 20 healthy controls (group III).[4]

Human papillomavirus (HPV)
HPV high risk is one if the most common sexually transmitted diseases. It is estimated that up to 85% of women will have been exposed to HPV in their life time. HPV high risk is usually harmless and will go away on its own. High risk HPV is associated with causing cervical cancer. HPV low risk causes genital warts and usually does not cause cervical cancer. Recently the CDC has recommended all eleven and twelve-year-old girls be vaccinated against HPV. Merck, the creators of the vaccine Gardisil, claims the vaccine can prevent certain strains of HPV. 13 of 100 strains of HPV are linked with causing cervical cancer.

Gardisil is marketed as only providing immunity for four of these strains. At $120 each, the three required does of Gardisil cost $360 per consumer, making it one of the most expensive vaccines on the market.[5] The vaccine does not prevent cervical cancer. The vaccine is to prevent the virus HPV. Cervical cancer testing and research is big money. The test is expensive and all women are encouraged to get tested yearly. At one time the herpes virus was suspecting of causing cervical cancer. In 1977, a virologist Harakd zur Hausen proposed the HPV virus was the cause of cervical cancer. When zur Hausen and his colleagues discovered that at least half the American adult population, and therefore half the adult women, had been infected by the virus, yet only one percent of women develop the cancer in their lifetimes, they began seeing a discrepancy.[6]

The best method of naturally immunizing is through breastfeeding. This should be followed by good hygiene and a diet of fresh vegetables, fruits, and whole grains. Parents who choose not to immunize with vaccines are within their legal rights. Children cannot be denied the right to public schooling simply because they are not vaccinated regardless of what school officials may try to make parents believe. If they receive money from the government they must respect the laws. According to the state parents live in they can simply file an exemption based on medical, philosophical, or religious beliefs. The decision to vaccinate or not vaccinate is personal. There is no federal law for vaccinations. Parents must do the research; after this is done they must do what feels right in their spirit, and ask for guidance. Vaccinations can also be avoided when traveling abroad. Many vaccines will be recommended when traveling to "high risk" areas. The yellow fever vaccine is commonly the only stated "mandatory" vaccine. Americans can refuse vaccines when traveling abroad. The World Health Organization in Geneva grants American citizens this right. Foreign Rules and Regulations, Part 71, Title 42 can be referenced when refusing vaccines while traveling abroad.

Are Allopathic doctors right for you and your family?

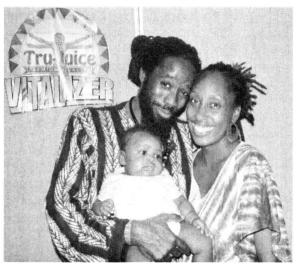

Courtesy of Kameela Abdul-Maajid,
Photography by Tioma Alison.

Four weeks after my son's birth I took him to a family physician for a check up. My spirit knew this was unnecessary, but I let other people persuade me. I thought things might go smoothly because this was a M.D. who prided himself in treating the mind, body, and spirit. So, I thought there would be no problems. I was wrong! I was given invalid information concerning the care of an intact and uncircumcised penis. I was also reprimanded for my choice not to vaccinate and refusing the PKU test. I did not feel the need to justify my choices. Nor, would I allow anyone to manipulate me into believing I was not a healer and the best knower concerning my child's health. Instead of confrontation I decided not to take my son back to the doctor. Pediatrician Dr. Robert Mendelsohn believes mother, father, and grandparents are the best doctors for children because they will allow the body to heal itself. The caregivers know and understand the child, not the doctors. He also suggests that the best way to keep your children healthy is to avoid doctors unless it is an emergency. The pediatrician serves as the recruiter for the medical profession. He indoctrinates the child from birth into a life long dependence on medical intervention. It begins with a succession of needles "well-baby check ups" and immunizations and then moves on to routine annual physical exams and endless treatment of minor ailments that would cure themselves if they were left alone.[7] Mendelsohn also points out, many doctors can and will report you to child services if you reject treatment he demands. This is one of the reasons I waived the PKU test. I am not sold on the accuracy of the test and would be obligated to follow the doctor's orders. As parents we have to be mindful of what we are getting ourselves into when we allow a doctor to become our child's PRIMARY health care provider. Parents who feel comfortable allowing their child to see pediatricians for non-emergencies should not be intimidated. They have the right to ask questions and refuse procedures. Many doctors abuse drugs such as antibiotics and will prescribe these drugs for common colds. Antibiotics and ear tubes are overly prescribed to children. Parents do not have to get the prescription filled. Antibiotics should be researched by the parents if they choose to use them before administering them to their children.

It is not easy for parents to watch children who are sick or uncomfortable. Due to the medicalized society of today, parents sometimes are quick to call the doctor if their child is not well. A 78-year-old Afrikan woman being interviewed by an anthropologist about health beliefs and practices of American ethnic groups said, "These white folks don' care nothin' 'bout you and me and they don' want to see us flerishin'. That's why so much of that medicine they always after us 'bout takin' is agains' us. These doctors ain nothin' but white folks, too".[8] Before coming to America, Afrikans did not go to physicians to treat ailments. They went to their diviners, healers, or went out and gathered herbs. They not only looked at the physical factors of the illness, but the social and spiritual factors as well. The chosen remedy was not to simply suppress the disease, but heal the mind, body, and soul. Toxic chemicals were not the only remedy for removing toxins from the body. Mrs. P, aged 82, also credited her long life and good health to the fact that she had always relied on her own herbal remedies, "My system ain't never been poisoned up by no medical doctor."[8]

Afrikan Medicinal Herbalism

Afrikans brought to the Americas and enslaved continued to use herbalism as a method of healing. Slaves did not have the same access to healthcare as their masters. They relied on herbal remedies. Many slaves were so skillful as natural healers, they were able to trade natural cures for their freedom. White southerners wrote slave remedies into their private recipe books even as they wrote laws curtailing the practice of enslaved doctors.[9] Europeans not only attempted to destroy the Afrikan's religion, but their traditional use of medicinal plants. Colonizers in Afrika did the same on the continent as well. The Afrikan's healing ways were seen as a threat. So, not only do many Afrikans reclaim their spirituality, but reclaim themselves as healers. Afrikans are juju, roots working, and healing peoples.

Ghana is known for its rich tradition of using Afrikan medicinal plants. 75% of Ghana's population uses traditional Afrikan medicine. In traditional Akan medicine the practice is very holistic, it is deeply rooted in traditional religion, with illness seen as a departure from the natural equilibrium.[10] Afrikans cannot forget their connection to the universe. Oneness with the universe is sometimes forgotten because of Eurocentricism. Many colonized and dispersed Afrikans have been led to believe god is outside of themselves. Therefore, they do not see god in the earth, water, plants, etc. Afrikans see god in everything and anything, this creates a balance. Interaction with the univere is reciprocal. So, the first step to healing is living with nature and trusting nature. Some people have no success with naturopathy because they do not trust nature. They trust only the synthetic which is man-made, Western medicine. They see the MD (medical deity) as a god, in fact worship him. Western medicine is a religion with the fanciest and biggest church building, where the tithes are high. Western medicine takes away from the body and does not replenish it. This is similar to the Afrikans relationship with the earth. They too must not take from the earth without replenishing it. Polluted air causes free radicals which can cause cancer. If the soil is depleted the plant life will lack vitamins and nutrients which results in disease of the body. Take the initiative to recycle, re-use plastics bags, and use natural home cleaning products. Herbs are no good if the soil they grow in is polluted. It is believed by Africans that where a plant grows also affects its spiritual powers (energy) to heal.[11]

The Yoruba of Nigeria also have a great respect for Afrikan medicinal herbalism. Orunmilla commonly known as the divination orisha (god) also revealed herbal medicine. The purpose of Yoruba is not merely to counteract the negative forces of disease in the human body, but also to achieve spiritual enlightenment and elevation which are the means of freeing the soul.[11] Afrikan parents on the path of holistic healing must look at the whole. What changes have taken place in the child's life?

• Relocation
• New school
• New friends
• Different energies in the home
• Diet change
• Emotional changes (depressed, withdrawn, anxious, etc)

Look at more than just the runny nose, fever, rash, and cough. Consider the child's emotional state too, not just the physical. Other people's emotions affect children also. Some people rarely get sick. This is not because they are the healthiest people in the world, but they simply have an innate way of transferring their negative energies and diseases to others. Afrikans are spiritually sensitive people. When the child is healed of her physical ailments look at the surroundings in the home and make changes as well. Use all the spiritual tools available when healing. Light a candle. Meditate on the ailment and listen to the spirit of the herbs. Ask the great mother healers for guidance, such as Yemaya and Oshun. If the child has a stomach ache parents can look to the orisha that governs the digestive area, Oshun. Her ewes (herbs) include cinnamon and chamomile. Both are excellent remedies for stomach aches. Our ancestors have left a tradition and a science of healing, embrace it, and claim it. Afrikans must move away from their colonized way of thinking. Healing is not just about giving a child cough syrup and antibiotics. Parents put on your all white clothes and go into your "kitchen laboratory" as Queen Afua calls it and let the spirit guide you. Use your sacred mortar and pestle to release the most high's healing energy from the herbs. Adama and Naomi Doumbia of Senegal consider the mortar and pestle a charm making tool:

> Over time a mortar builds up a high charge of nyama from the medicines and herbs we prepare in it. The mortar and pestle symbolize the feminine and masculine principles, together representing the sacred act of creation. When we bring the mortar and pestle together, we are unifying the transcendent with the immanent. We raise our pestles high in the air, calling the heavens, and rhythmically stroke the pestle into the mortar, the womb of the earth.[12]

When children are sick it can be a daunting experience. However, parents can find joy when they are healing with the power of the spirit. What negative energy or disease can defeat joy and laughter? Het Heru and Oshun are healing goddesses that remind parents to put a smile on their faces even through difficult times. The parents are the child's first and primary healers. During slavery, mothers were usually not able to tend to their children when sick. They were working the fields or tending to the master's children. Children were usually tended to by the elders. Many white slave owners believed Afrikan mothers were incompetent and could not be trusted. In *Working Cures: Healing, Health, and Power on Southern Slave Plantations*, Sharla M. Fett states:

> Samuel Cartwright wove the theme of maternal deficit into his litany of the failings of the Afrikan Americans as race. He charged that slave mothers with sick children deviated from the natural maternal impulses of white women, "They let their children suffer and die, or unmercifully abuse them," he wrote. Linking the depravity of slave mothers to the racialized maternal bounty of white mistresses, he credited the survival of black children to the intervention of southern mistresses with their nursery rules. Charles Lyell, too, sketched "negro mothers" as a group "often so ignorant or indolent, that they can not be trusted to keep awake and administer medicine to their own children," hence creating the need for the vigilance of their mistresses.[9]

Physicians today also try to strip the mother's right to heal their children, and make their own decisions regarding their child's healthcare. Parents have the right to nurse their children in a holistic fashion. They do not have to apologize for using herbs, refusing vaccinations, and tests. When healing, have the confidence to meditate on the ailment and look at the whole picture. Examine which ailments, herbs, oils, and physiological factors relate to the Abosom/Neter/Orisha/Loa. Former slave and herb doctor George White explained, "Dere's a root for ev'y disease an' I can cure just about anything, but you have to talk wid God an' ask him to help out."[9] Afrikan slaves of the Diaspora practicing Santeria and Candomble went out to the forest and honored the Yoruba deity Osain/Osanyin with libations before gathering herbs.

Herb	Uses	Orisha	How To Use
Aloe Vera	Burns, mosquito bites, pinworms, laxative	Yemaya	Apply gel directly to skin
Anise	Gas, cough, mucus clearing,	Oshun	Tea, capsule, spice
Basil	Cold, flu, fever, constipation	Oshun, Yemaya, Obatala	Tea, capsule, spice
Black Elder Flower and Berries	Flu, fever, sore throat	Oshun, Obatala	Tea wash, salve, oil
Calendula	Eye wash for irritated eyes, skin irritations, wounds, scrapes,	Oya, Oshun	Tea, herbal wash, oil, capsule, herbal bath
Catnip	Calming, indigestion, makes the child sweat	Oshun	Tea, capsule
Cayenne	Flu, external bleeding	Shango	Capsule, directly on skin
Chamomile	Anxiety, restless, stomach, gas, colic, sleep aid,	Elegba	Tea, salve, tincture, poultice, capsule, oil,

99

Herb	Uses	Orisha	How To Use
	constipation		herbal wash
Cinnamon	Nausea, Vomiting, chills, gas	Oshun	Tea, capsule, oil, spice
Clove	Teething, toothaches, gas	Oshun	Tea, oil
Echinacea	Cods, flu, inflam mations, wounds, fever, bites	Oshun	Tea, salve, tincture, poultice, capsule, oil, ear drops
Fennel	Colic, indigestion, gas, coughs, nausea	Elegba	Tea, spice, capsule
Garlic	Parasites, cold, flu, fever, earaches	Yemaya, Ogun	Tea, salve, tincture, poultice, capsule, oil, ear drops, spice, paste
Ginger	Cold, flu, fever, congestion, chills, sore throat	Orunmilla, Oshun	Spice, capsule, paste, tea, herbal bath, herbal wash
Lemon Balm	Body aches, fever, calming, cold sores, gas, anxiety, crying	Elegba	Tea, salve, tincture, poultice, capsule, oil, herbal steam, herbal bath
Licorice	Cough, laxative, mucous clearer, congestion, sore throat	Elegba	Tea, capsule, tincture, spice
Mullein	Earaches, skin	Oya	Tea, salve,

100

Herb	Uses	Orisha	How To Use
	irritations, coughs, bronchitis, cold, flu		tincture, poultice, capsule, oil, ear drops
Peppermint	Gas, colic	Oshun	Tea, tincture, oil, capsule
Plantain	Bites, stings, wounds, inflammations	Oya	Tea, salve, tincture, poultice, capsule, oil, ear drops, herbal wash, herbal bath
Sage	Flu, colds, sore throat, diarrhea	Orunmilla, Obatala	Spice, tea, herbal wash
Slippery Elm	Wounds, diaper rash, skin irritations, nutritious whole food, diarrhea indigestion	Elegba	Tea, salve, tincture, poultice, capsule, oil, herbal wash
Thyme	Whooping cough, lice, bronchitis, wounds	Elegba	Tea, capsule, herbal wash
Yarrow	Colds, flu, burns, cuts, wounds	Oshun, Yemaya	Tea, salve, tincture, poultice, capsule, oil

How to use herbs

Salves

Choose your herbs. Decide how many parts you would like to you use. If you are making a small amount, use a half teaspoon or half tablespoon as your part. Use a cup or more for larger amounts.

- Add the herbs to a crock pot.
- Cover your herbs with olive oil, a half inch to an inch.
- Heat the herbs for three hours.
- Let the herbs cool.
- Strain your oil and herbs with a strainer lined with cheesecloth.
- For small preparations begin with adding a 1/2 oz of beeswax to the oil. Many find it easier to grate the beeswax. To check the consistency, place a small amount on a spoon and place in the refrigerator for 3-5 minutes. If it is too soft add more beeswax to the pot.
- Pour mixture in a dark container.

* If you want to make an ointment use the same directions, only use less beeswax.

Herbal Steams

- Make an herbal tea in a pot with the herbs of your choice.
- Add boiled water to a bowl or basin.
- Drape a towel over the head and lean over the steam, but be careful not to get to close.
- Breathe in for up to 5–10 minutes.

* This is great for congestion or breathing difficulties.

Herbal Baths

- Place herbs of choice in a muslin bag or piece of cloth.
- Tie the cloth on the faucet where it hangs in the flowing water. When done place the bag in the bath water. If you would like the herbs to be stronger make a tea and pour in the water.

Poultices

- Smash herbs and place on skin.

- When using dry herbs, add water. No water is needed if the herbs are fresh. Place the herbs directly on the skin or use cheese cloth or any thin piece of cloth.
- If using cloth, place cloth on skin, add herbs, and place another piece of cloth over the herb. Cloth is usually used with herbs that may irritate the skin. A hot water bottle is optional.

Herbal Teas

There are multiple ways to make an herbal tea. The tea can be steeped, made into an infusion, or decoction. To steep your tea place a tea bag, tea ball, or loose herbs in boiling water for 10 - 20 minutes. A medicinal tea is normally made using one ounce of herbs to 2 cups of water.[13]

Tea Infusions

- Boil water in tea or cooking pot.
- Place herbs in the pot of water.
- Pour boiling water in the pot.
- Cover and let it sit 15-20 minutes. You can let it sit for up to eight hours, depending on the desired strength. The tea can sit in a glass- covered jar.
- Strain the tea.

Tea Decoctions

A decoction is made by boiling herbs and roots in a pot. This is more concentrated than an infusion.

- Add herbs and water to a pot.
- Cover the herbs and bring to a boil.
- Turn the heat down to a low simmer for up to 30 minutes.

Herbal Wash

Make the desired tea. Use a wash cloth to apply the tea to the body.

Paste

Paste can be made with herbs for the skin using raw honey or water.

Herbal Oils
- Add desired herbs to a jar.
- Add enough oil to fill the jar. Oils such as olive, sesame, or almond can be used.
- Cover the jar.
- Store away from direct sunlight for three days up to two weeks depending on the herbs.
- Squeeze the remaining oil from your cheese cloth
- Add vitamin E capsule.
- Pour mixture in a glass container.

Syrups
Syrups are usually made using either honey or glycerin.
Make a tea or decoction using the herbs of choice.
- Strain the tea or decoction.
- Use a ½ cup of the tea or decoction and two cups of honey or glycerin.

Tinctures
- Fresh or dried herbs can be used. Fresh herbs should be chopped. Dried herbs should be grinded.
- Use 100-proof Vodka or 200-proof grain alcohol.
- Herbalist, Aviva Jill Romm, recommends placing about two ounces of plant material in a pint jar.[14]
- Pour the alcohol to the top of the jar.
- Seal the jar and place it in a dark room or drawer.
- Shake the jar every one or two days for 2-4 weeks.
- After the two week period strain the mixture using a strainer lined with cheese cloth.
- Remove the remaining liquid from the cheese cloth by squeezing it.
- Store the liquid in a dark glass jar or tincture bottle and label.
- Keep tinctures made with alcohol out of the reach of children!

Herbal dosages for Children

Children should not be given the same amount of herbs as adults.

104

Clark's rule is a method of determining the dosage for children. Most standard herbal dosages are for 150 pound adults. To determine a child's dosage divide the child's weight by 150 Ex: 50/150 = 1/3 The children's dosage will be 1/3 of the adult dosage.

Lesley Tierra, L.aAc., AHG author of *A Kid's Herb Book: for children of all ages*, summarizes Clark's rule, a standing formula for prescribing children's dosages for herbal teas:[13]

Weight	Herb Tea
Up to 5 pounds	1 tablespoon
5 – 15 pounds	2 tablespoon
16-35 pounds	¼ cup
36-65 pounds	½ cup
66-80 pounds	¾ cup
81-110 pounds	1 cup (adult dose)

Mother and Father are the child's primary care givers
My first real test as a healer for my son was when he was seventeen-months-of-age. He had a fever close to 104 degrees in the early A.M. There was no cough, sneezing, congestion, or mucus. A few days earlier he had a slight temperature. I assumed he was teething. He was only cranky and tired. I placed onions in his socks to bring down the temperature. Onions were also placed in gauze and placed around his forehead and chest. He was sponged down with an herbal wash of lemon balm, cat nip, echinacea, and ginger. Three times a day he was given an herbal tincture with echinacea, peppermint leaf, elder flowers, yarrow flowers, and catnip. He was also given plenty of fluids, including an herbal tea of lemon balm and catnip. By 7:30 P.M. the fever was gone. My son slept in the bed with me that night. I woke up around 2:30 A.M. and he was cold. I took his auxiliary (arm pit) temperature. It was 93.5 degrees. I became scared. All I could think of was hypothermia. I woke him. His pulse and respiration was checked. I looked for symptoms of lethargy. This was followed by checking his eyes for pupil dilation. I checked his rectal temperature just to make sure the auxiliary temperature was not off. The temperature was 96 degrees or so. He was sleeping by now. During the whole event he simply wanted to sleep. I felt

better with the new temperature. I am not sure if the sweating out of the fever caused the low temperature or my initial temperature was wrong. It could have just been that waking temperatures are usually low. I lit my altar that night and asked for guidance. By the A.M. he was back to his normal self. 98.6 degrees is the body's average temperature. However, body temperature can vary from person to person. A temperature of 101.5 is considered to be a fever. Fever is not totally understood. Many believe it is the body's way of helping to fight infection. A temperature up to 102 degrees does not have to be lowered if the child is functioning as normal. Fever reaching 101.5 in infants particularly three months or younger can be cause for alarm. Temperatures below 95 degrees are also cause for alarm. Low temperatures can cause hypothermia. Children can become extremely cold and lethargic. Children under four-years-of-age usually have their temperatures taken rectally. The armpit is also option. However, it can be up to two degrees lower than a rectal temperature. Ear thermometers have been known to read to high. Children five years and older can have their temperatures taken orally. Use digital thermometers to avoid mercury exposure.

Many illnesses or ailments can be cared for by the parents. Children can also can receive routine home healthcare or receive it in addition to a naturopaths or physician's care. Height, weight, glands, nose, neck, eyes, and skin can be checked to make sure the child is in optimal health. The height and weight allows parent to monitor growth developments or sudden changes. Checking the child's glands in the neck area can alert parents of infection if swollen. Having the child perform side to side neck movements can determine if they have stiff neck. Mucus in the nose can be a sign of infection. Clear or white mucus can be a sign of colds or allergy. Green or yellow mucus is a sign of possible sinus or respiratory infection. Watery, irritated, or dull eyes can be signs of illness. Healthy children usually do not have dark rings around the eyes. Bulging eyes can be a sign of thyroid problems. Eyes that do not dilate properly can signal head injury or other conditions. The skin should be checked for rashes, bruises, lumps, cuts, and other abnormalities.

Optional and Suggested Medical Supplies for Evaluating Your Child's Health

Otoscope

An otoscope can be useful in detecting ear infections, excess wax/mucus and objects. Home otoscopes are reasonably priced, but are not the same quality as the physician grade. The eardrum should be transparent. If it looks abnormal or inflamed this could be signs of infection. Also look for puss.

Stethoscope

A stethoscope allows you to listen to the child's heart beat and lungs.

Blood Pressure Cuff

A blood pressure cuff allows parents to check children's blood pressure.

Pen Light

Parents have the ability to look at the child's mouth, throat, and eyes. Check for redness, swelling, white spots and yeast in the mouth, and throat area.

CPR and Vital sign knowledge

Parents and caregivers should have CPR (cardiopulmonary resuscitation) training. CPR can save children's lives. Most CPR classes teach mouth to mouth resuscitation, cardiac emergencies, choking, first aid, and poison prevention. CPR and first aid is taught at institutions such as the American Red Cross. Vitals signs are the signs of life. They can be checked by temperature, pulse, respiration, and blood pressure.

Respiration Rate

Respiration rate is breaths per minute.

Blood Pressure

Blood Pressure is the force of blood flowing through the arteries.

Pulse

The pulse can be found on the side of the neck, carotid pulse. Finding the pulse on the neck of young children can be difficult. It can also be found inside the arm above the elbow, brachial pulse. A stopwatch or watch with a second hand can be used. The tips of the index and middle fingers are placed on the pulse. Begin counting when the clock hits zero. Count until 60 seconds.

The University of Nebraska Medical Center has defined normal vital signs for children.[15]

Age Group	Pulse Rate	Respiration Rate	Blood Pressure Range
Babies	120 - 150	30 - 60	Usually do not measure
2 to 6 years old	90 - 120	20 - 35	80/75 to 110/75
Children	85 - 100	18 - 25	75/40 to 120/75
Teenage	70 - 100	16 - 25	85/45 to 130/85
Adult	60 - 100	12 - 20	100/50 to 139/89

Source: University of Nebraska Medical Center
http://www.unmc.edu/nursing/careers/nurse_facts.htm

Preparing For Emergencies
Parents and caregivers should keep emergency contact numbers on the refrigerator and phone. If the fire department or paramedics have to enter the home and remove family members from the home an emergency contact can be called immediately. Cell phones should have the emergency contacts stored under ICE (In Case of Emergency).

Poison Prevention
Poisonous products should be kept out of the home or placed on high shelves out of reach. Most poisonous substances in the home are commercial home cleaners. Use natural home cleaners instead. Parents and caregivers should have activated charcoal and Ipecac available in the home. Ipecac is being used less, because if used incorrectly it can cause harm. Never use Ipecac unless told to do so by Poison Control. Ipecac is to never be used when the child has swallowed something caustic such as commercial cleaning products. This can cause the chemical to burn the child's throat when vomiting. Activated charcoal absorbs some poisons. Before attempting to do anything call Poison Control, NOT the 911 operator. The Poison Control Number is 1-800-222-1222.

911
Teach children at a very young age how to dial 911. Even if they do not talk well, a phone left off the hook will send emergency personnel to the home. Many children have called 911 for adults and have saved lives.

Fire Emergencies
Place tot finder stickers on children's bedroom windows. Every family should have an escape plan. Parents should conduct periodic fire drills. The family should be out of the home within three minutes. Children must know the best way to get out. They must also know when to stay put. Working smoke detectors in the home are a must. Check them frequently.

Fire Safety Tips Children Should Know

- Doors should not be opened if the knobs are hot.
- Check under the crack of the door to see if smoke is present. If smoke is present do not open the door. Block the smoke and heat with blankets and clothes.
- Clothes or sheets can be placed over the mouth to avoid smoke inhalation. Wet cloth works best.
- Keep low to the ground where there is less smoke.
- Do not look for pets.

- Do not hide in places such as under the bed, closets, or behind dressers. Rescue personnel must be able to locate the children.
- Children should know how to unlock doors, windows, and pull out screens in case of emergencies only.
- If clothes catch on fire, roll around until fire is put out.
- Children are not to go back into the house once out.

First Aid
It is essential to have a first aid kit in the home. It can be purchased or made at home. The kit should contain scissors, gauze, medical tape, tweezers, bandages, hot/cold pack, and alcohol wipes. Herbal supplies may include:

Supplies	Use
Activated Charcoal	Can be used for poisoning. **Call Poison Control before using**.
Aloe Vera	A natural laxative, soothes cuts, burns, and scrapes.
Cayenne	Stops internal bleeding.
Echinacea	Is an antibiotic. Helps relieve colds and fever.
Ginger	Useful for colds, flu, and fever.
Goldenseal	A natural antibiotic. Can be used as paste, added to poultices, or used as powder in bandages.
Herbal Salves made of calendula, comfrey, echinacea, lavender, St. Johns wart, plantain, etc.	Can be used for cuts, bruises, scrapes, diaper rash and skin irritations.
Ipecac	Can be used for poisoning. **Call Poison Control before using**.
Peppermint	Useful for gas pains and stomach aches.
Plantain leaf	Soothes and heals scratches, cuts, and bites. Can be used as a

	poultice.
Tea tree oil	An antibiotic and antifungal.
Valerian	Can be used as a sedative.
Yarrow	Stops external bleeding.

Nutrition

I encourage pregnant mothers to eat plenty of fruits and vegetables, so the baby's palate will be receptive to healthy foods and herbs. If mothers want green babies they must eat green. When my son was a year old, he was no stranger to raw pepper, garlic, onions, tomatoes, and green leafy vegetables. He was exposed to these foods in the womb. Mothers and fathers must establish a healthy lifestyle prior to conception. They must be healthy emotionally and spiritually. Release hurt, misgivings, and guilt caused by mates or others. Do not pass these legacies to the next generation. Afrikans need healthy sperm fertilizing healthy eggs.

There are many great food enhancers and super foods for children. A healthy diet is key to optimal health. When children begin eating, emphasize vegetables and fruits first. Feeding too much starch can cause children to become addicted to the taste of sugar. Children should only eat whole grains, do not feed them white bread, white rice, and other bleached white products. Instead of feeding toddlers snacks such as cookies, give them raw sliced tomatoes, celery, cucumbers, and fruits. If parents put starch first, so will the child. Create a palate in alignment with green and raw foods. Feed children the foods which are in season for optimal nutrition. Keep assorted fruits, veggie plates, and trail mixes available for children to snack on during the day. Parents are in control of the child's taste buds. Vegetables can be steamed instead of boiled to preserve nutrients. Give the child at least one raw food meal a day if possible. Zakhah's, *The Joy Of Living Live: A Raw Food Journey* has plenty of ethnic raw food dishes from around the world.

Quick Raw Food Snacks for Children:

- Avocadoes wrapped in lettuce.

111

- Celery sticks topped with nut/seed butter and raisins.
- Raw okra, corn, and tomatoes. This can be seasoned with liquid aminos or Tamari sauce. Spike can also be used.
- Raw corn on the cob seasoned with spike and dairy-free margarine.
- Fruit Salad

Avoid processed foods as much as possible. If you do buy them read labels carefully. Avoid preservatives, additives, dyes, aspartame, sodium nitrate, potassium bromate, high fructose corn syrup, and monosodium glutamate (MSG).

Monosodium glutamate (MSG)

MSG is a flavor enhancer. It is also toxic. MSG has been associated with attention deficit disorder (ADD), and endocrine brain disorders. MSG is often disguised on labels under names such as: textured protein, natural flavorings, hydrolyzed protein, hydrolyzed plant protein, hydrolyzed vegetable protein, stock, broth, natural beef flavoring, natural chicken flavoring, yeast extract, hydrolyzed oat flour, malt extract, calcium caseinate, and sodium caseinate.

BHA and BHT

Preservatives such as Butylated hydroxyanisole (BHA) and butylated hydroxytoluene (BHT), commonly used in cereals many children eat everyday, causes cancer in rats.

Potassium Bromate

Every country except for the Unites States and Japan has banned potassium bromate. It is commonly used in breads. Potassium Bromate was found to have carcinogenic affects in rats. The incidences of tumor-bearing animals were very high in both control and treated groups of both sexes. This phenomenon resulted from the high incidences of tumors of kidney, testis, peritoneum, thyroid, pituitary, mammary gland and spleen.[16]

112

Food Coloring

Many foods have synthetic food coloring. The most common dyes seen on labels are red and yellow dyes. Food coloring is an allergen and causes cancer in rats. It is also linked with behavioral problems such as ADD. In urban communities especially, you see children drinking "forties", high fructose syrup dyed with Red 40. These same children usually have behavioral problems. One Red 40 study states:

> Female rats were given Red 40 during lactation and gestation. Parental animals were evaluated for weight and food consumption, and females for reproductive success. The offspring were assessed on a series of tests using the Cincinnati Psychoteratogenicity Screening Test Battery. Additional measures were weight, food consumption, physical landmarks of development, and brain weight. Red-40 significantly reduced reproductive success, parental and offspring weight, brain weight, survival, and female vaginal patency development. Behaviorally, R40 produced substantially decreased running wheel activity, and slightly increased postweaning open-field rearing activity. Overall, R40 produced evidence of both physical and behavioral toxicity in developing rats at doses of up to 10% of the diet.[17]

Aspartame (Nutrasweet®)

Aspartame is a sugar substitute. It is toxic. Children who display symptoms of ADD and ADHD will have worsened behavior. Aspartame is related to causing cancer, diabetes, seizures, anxiety, birth defects, brain tumors, and brain cell damage.

Sodium Nitrate

Sodium Nitrate is commonly used to preserve packaged meat products. It is a carcinogen which can cause cancer.

High Fructose Corn Syrup

113

High fructose corn syrup is a form of sugar derived from genetically modified corn. High fructose corn syrup in rats causes liver damage, reproductive failure, anemia, copper deficiency, high cholesterol, and heart enlargement. High fructose corn syrup is commonly found in juice, soda, cereal, ketchup, snacks, and much more. Parents can avoid high fructose syrup in processed foods by shopping at natural food stores. White sugar should also be avoided. Raw sugar, pure maple syrup, honey, and molasses are better options for sweeteners. However, use sweeteners in moderation. They are not always necessary. These sweeteners too can be unhealthy if used excessively.

Genetically Modified Foods (GMOs) and Pesticides

Buy organic food when possible to avoid GMOs and pesticides. Genetically modified foods are those which genes have been altered. A gene from another species is sometimes added. Sometimes a gene is subtracted from the plant. Corn is a crop genetically modified often. Is corn that has the genes of another vegetable species still corn? What are the consequences of the pollen from a genetically modified plants invading fields where other non–gmo foods are grown? What affects does this have on the eco-system? Are we in danger of losing our natural plant foods? Will the foods nutritional content be jeopardized? The dangers and lasting affects of GMOs on the environment have not been thoroughly studied.

Pesticides sprayed onto fruits and vegetables are toxic. Pesticides also decrease the nutritional value of foods. In a review of 41 studies from around the world, organic crops were shown to have significantly higher levels of vitamin C, magnesium, iron, and phosphorous. Spinach, lettuce, cabbage, and potatoes showed particularly high levels of minerals.[18] Do not spray yards and gardens with weed killers, chemical pesticides, and herbicides. Do not let your child play in grass sprayed with herbicides or pesticides. Shoes should not be worn in the home. They can bring filth, herbicides, and pesticides in the home. Children spend a lot of time on the floors and place their fingers in their mouths. These chemicals are poisonous. Pesticides cause neurological damage, behavioral disorders, developmental disorders, cancer, increased risk of childhood leukemia, and low birth weight infants. Children are especially at risk because of their immature immune systems. Be aware that their bodies are still in the developmental stages. Children need the best foods available. A recent study in the journal of Environmental Health Perspectives found that pesticide levels dropped immediately when children started eating the organic foods.[18]

Super Supplements
Omega 3 6 9 Essential Fatty Acids
Fatty acids are essential for fetal and infant brain development. They boost the immune system, promote healing, improve vision, and support the heart. Vegetarian Omega 3 6 9 formulas can be purchased. Add essential fatty acids to smoothies, salads, and cereal.

Slippery Elm
Slippery Elm is a nutritious food that is an antioxidant and detoxifier. It promotes cellular, intestinal, and stomach health. Slippery Elm can be added to hot cereals and smoothies.

Wheat Germ
Wheat germ is high in iron and potassium especially. It also contains B complex, vitamin E, protein, magnesium, lecithin, zinc, phosphorus, and calcium. Wheat germ supports the immune system, provides energy and supports heart function. Wheat germ can be added to cereals, smoothies, soy yogurts, and vegetables.

Nutritional Yeast
Nutritional yeast is high in protein and B vitamins, including B-12. Nutritional yeast can be added to popcorn, sprinkled over pasta dishes, and added to vegetables.

Flaxseed Oil
Flaxseed oil contains Omega 3 fatty acids and alpha-linolenic acid. Improves immune system health, prevents heart disease, and supports nervous system. Add to salads, vegetables, non-dairy milks, and smoothies. Do not heat flaxseed oil.

Blackstrap Molasses

Blackstrap Molasses is high in iron, calcium, and potassium. It can be added to smoothies and non-dairy milks.

Spirulina
Spirulina is a blue green algae high in chlorophyll, protein, and vitamin B-12. It can be added to water, juice, and smoothies.

Wheatgrass
Wheatgrass contains B, C, E, and A vitamins. It is also a good source of iron, calcium, magnesium, and is rich in chlorophyll. It is an excellent detoxifier, improves hemoglobin counts, and boosts the immune system. Wheatgrass can be added to water, juice, and smoothies. Fresh wheatgrass can be drunk alone for children who can tolerate it.

Super Foods
Nuts and Seeds
Nuts and seeds are highly nutritious. They contain the fats that are essential for the child's development, omega fatty acids. Nuts and seeds also are high in protein. Sesame seeds, sunflower seeds, cashews, flaxseeds, and walnuts are especially nutritious. Nuts and seeds can be eaten by themselves or ground in a blender or grinder to make seed or nut milks. After grinding add water to the blender. The milk will have to be blended and strained a few times. Bananas or maple syrup can be used as sweeteners. Ground seeds and nuts can also be added to smoothies. For a nutritious snack give children trail mix.

Avocados
Avocados are a great source of fatty acids, oleic acid, vitamin E, potassium, lutein, carotenoids, and B vitamins. Avocados can be eaten as is or added to sandwiches, salads, and burritos.

Sprouts
When foods are sprouted and eaten raw the nutritional factor drastically increases. The sprouting process makes it easier for the body to absorb nutrients. Eating foods raw is best; however some foods are not easily digested raw. Sprouting makes it possible to eat many foods raw such as beans, sesame seeds, fenugreek, chickpeas, rice, sunflower seeds, and lentils. Alfalfa, broccoli,

arugula, wheat grass, clover, barley, oat, wheat, and kamut, can also be sprouted. The sprouting process is simple. Wide mouth jars with cheese cloth or a sprout cover is used. Sprouting bags and trays are also available. Depending on the seed it may have to be soaked anywhere from 4-12 hours. The seeds are then drained and place in a container. They are then rinsed and drained twice a day. After a day or two the seeds will sprout. The sprouting process can take 2-10 days depending on the seed. Sprouting can be fun and educational for children. Let them sprout their own foods. Sprouts can be eaten as is or added to salads or wraps.

Millet
Millet is a staple food in Afrika. It was eaten by the ancestors. Millet is high in iron, protein, B vitamins, potassium, fiber, magnesium, and phosphorus. Of all the grains millet is one of the least allergenic. Home-made millet cereal is an excellent food for infants; it is very easy to digest. Millet can be used as a side dish instead of rice. Use 1 part millet and 2 parts water. To achieve a creamier consistency use 1 part millet and 3 parts water. Millet can be used to make breads, stews, cereals, pancakes, and much more.

Quinoa
Quinoa is a complete protein. It contains all 8 essential amino acids. It is also high in copper, manganese, and riboflavin. Quinoa can be added to vegetable stir - frys, stews, salads, or eaten in place of rice. Use 1 part quinoa and 2 parts liquid.

Kale
Kale is a good source of fiber, manganese, vitamin A, vitamin C, lutein, and calcium. It is highly nutritious and a cancer fighting food. Kale can be steamed or boiled in a small amount of water. It is also delicious raw. Raw kale can be marinated in an olive oil, minced garlic, and tamari sauce. It can also be marinated in natural Italian dressing.

Juicing
A great way to make sure children get their daily fruits and vegetables is through juicing. Many nutrients are lost during the heating of foods. Juicing provides the live enzymes, minerals, and

vitamins needed for optimal health. Dead food is not going to maintain the health of a living body. The key to keeping children out of hospitals and doctor's offices is to keep them healthy. Natural healing methods do not always work effectively when consuming a toxic diet. So, preventative medicine must be used. Children can sometimes be picky and eat small portions. Juicing can alleviate these problems. Juicing provides a way to add antioxidants to the diet too. Wheat grass, a powerful antioxidant can be juiced at home. Fruits such as berries and apples can be juiced with wheatgrass to mask the taste for children.

Juicing requires a juicer. Do some research before investing in one. The best juicers usually are expensive. It may be wise to invest in a cheaper juicer initially. So, if you decide to stop juicing you will not have wasted too much money. Fruits and vegetables should be washed carefully. Organic is always best. Organic foods are higher in nutrients. Fruit and vegetable juices should be consumed within twenty-four hours. Store juices to be used later carefully. Clean your juicer after each use.

There are a variety of vegetables and fruits great for juicing such as: kale, spinach, broccoli, wheatgrass, apples, oranges, dandelion, cabbage, beets, carrots, grapes, parsley, grapefruit, mangoes, papaya, berries, lemons, pears, lettuce, and much more.

Recipe ideas

Carrots, Apple, and Celery
4 carrots
1 apple
1 celery stick

Carrots and Spinach
½ cup – 1 cup of spinach
6 carrots

Kale, Apple, and Cucumber
½ cup – 1 cup of kale
2 apples
1 cucumber

118

Have fun experimenting and creating your own recipes.

Smoothies are also great meals in a drink. Smoothies make it easy to add supplements such as wheat germ, chlorophyll, wheatgrass, blackstrap molasses,` and spirulina. Nut and seed butters can be added for creating a high protein smoothie. Smoothies are usually made by adding frozen fruits to non-dairy milks. Bananas provide an added thickness. Some great fruits to use are berries, mangos, papaya, oranges, and peaches.

Is the vegan diet safe for children?
The vegan diet is safe for children. However, it can be unsafe too. Any diet can be unsafe. Most meat-eating and junk food diets are dangerous. But parents with sick vegan children are more likely to be scrutinized and physicians will sometimes blame the vegan diet. This rarely happens with meat-eating children. In some extreme cases vegan parents have been reported to children services. Vegan parents must make sure their children are eating a whole foods diet, not just a vegan diet. Vegan families do not eat animal flesh or animal by-products. There are many foods I will not eat that are considered vegan. I do not like to label myself as simply a vegan, but will use it for clarity sake. I prefer holistic eating or a Maat diet. The laws of Maat encourage us to not pollute the land, regard all life and animals as sacred, only eat your fair share, and keep the water pure. Livestock production uses a lot of land that could be used to grow nutritious foods. A large amount of water and energy is wasted to support livestock production. Nearby water sources are sometimes polluted with livestock waste. The vegan diet does more than just keep people healthy, but it is also healthy for the environment.

Vegan children eating a whole foods diet are less likely to get sick compared to their non-whole food and meat eating counterparts. Critics will argue plants have protein, but not in large enough amounts. Most foods contain protein. Some plant based foods extremely high in protein are beans, nuts, seeds, kamut, quinoa, sea vegetables (kelp, duce, Irish moss, nori, spirulina), and tofu. Children simply need a varied diet to meet their protein and caloric needs. The SAD (Standard American Diet) has too much

119

protein which can have unhealthy affects and prevent absorption of some vitamins and minerals. Vegan children can meet there B-12 needs though supplements and fortified foods such as cereal and non-dairy milks. Nutritional yeast and spirulina contain vitamin B-12, but do not rely on them solely. Iron sources include dark leafy green vegetables, beans, nuts, seeds, dried fruits, blackstrap molasses and whole grains. A multi-vitamin is recommended as a supplement for children because the soil foods are grown in is sometimes depleted of many nutrients. Non-organic foods have even less nutrients and minerals.

Dairy is not necessary in a child's diet. Most Afrikans are lactose intolerant. Peggy O'mara author of the book *Natural Family Living* states:

> All mammal species, of course, produce milk as a complete food to nourish their young until they are weaned. After weaning, most mammals do not ever again drink milk. The exceptions are Hindus, Europeans, and Americans, who drink cow's milk. A sizeable majority of traditional cultures in the world do not drink milk, including most Asian and Afrikan populations.[1]

Children can receive calcium through dark leafy green vegetables, broccoli, almonds, okra, and blackstrap molasses. Collard greens are especially high in calcium. Cow's milk can be problematic because it contains a high amount of protein which can cause a calcium drain. Dairy also can affect iron absorption. Cow's milk also contains puss (white blood cells) caused by the machines that pump the cows milk. Non-organic milk contains antibiotics and the recombinant Bovine Growth Hormone (rBGH). Do you ever wonder why children's bodies develop earlier today? Children should be taken to farms. They should see where meat and milk come from. Let them see farm animals eat vegetation, not meat. Allow children to go to farms where plant foods are grown. Many inner city children do not know where the food comes from. It simply comes from the market in their eyes. Children should experience planting and growing foods inside and outside the home, or the community garden. They need to feel the soil in their hands. This establishes a connection to the earth.

Children should also stay away from white refined sugar which drains the body of its vitamins and nutrients. Sugar is very addictive and can cause behavior problems. Caffeine has the same affect. This toxic combination can be found in soda and carbonated drinks. Children should be drinking plenty of water and 100 percent juice instead. Water that has not refrigerated is easier on the body and easier to drink. Children need eight glasses of water a day. They are very active and can dehydrate fairly easy. Children should not drink water packaged in the opaque type plastic bottles. These bottles are made of Polyvinyl Chloride (PVC), which leaches into the water. PVCs are toxic. Many school age children do not get the adequate amount of water they need during the school day. Send your children to school with a water bottle if they are not homeschooled. Let the teacher know your child will be drinking water through out the day. Vegan parents should also leave some vegan treats with the teacher. Many classrooms have events that are not always planned where the children will receive foods or snacks. This will enable the child to not feel left out. Make it very clear to the teachers and staff that your child is a vegan and should not be given any foods besides the ones that the child brings. Vegan children attending birthday parties can still have birthday cake and ice cream. Parents can make a vegan cake or buy them from the major health food store chains. Dairy-free ice cream can also be purchased.

Vegan lunchbox ideas

- Soups, stews, and chili in a thermos
- Cold pasta salad (noodles, tomatoes, broccoli, cucumber, peppers, and Italian dressing)
- Burritos made with beans, rice, lettuce, and tomato
- Pitas stuffed with lettuce, tomato, sprouts, couscous, and avocado
- Hummus and pita bread
- Sunflower seed butter on whole wheat or sprouted bread
- Falafels, cucumber, lettuce, tomato, and tahini stuffed in a pita

121

6 - Toxic Free Home & Sustainable Living

Home Environment

The home should be reflective of the family's culture and spirit. Children should have a sense of culture and pride. This starts in the home. Children should know the home is a spiritual place that should be respected. No shoes should be allowed in the home. Keep dirt and filth from your temple. Children spend a lot of time on the floors.

Fill your house with inspirational sounds. When I was in Ghana, West Afrika everywhere I went I heard music. My videotapes of the trip have their own theme songs. What would you like the theme songs of your home to be? Choose something culturally and spiritually enriching. Children should be familiar with Afrikan drums and sounds very early in life. The aromas in the home should be therapeutic for the family. Incense can be burned in the home to please the senses and dispel negative energy. Frankincense and myrrh are excellent for smudging and purifying the home. Cinnamon brooms are great to have in the home. They can be found in many natural food chains, especially during the December holidays. The smell of cinnamon permeating the home during the winter solstice is absolutely delightful. Walls should have pictures of the family and ancestors. It is great to have Afrikan heroes on the wall such as Malcolm X, Kwame Nkrumah, John Henrik Clarke, Queen Nzinga, Assata Shakur, Harriet Tubman, John Coltrane, and Stephen Bantu Biko. Afrikan tapestry and fabrics are a nice accent to the home. Wooden Afrikan carvings, sculptures, paintings and masks should also be placed around the home. Set up mini altars in different places in the home representative of the elements. These can include: candles, rocks, water, plants, and incense.

The home should be free of clutter. Things no longer used should be thrown out. A cluttered house literally clutters the mind. It is hard for children to concentrate surrounded by clutter. The house should be kept clean and tidy. Rooms with a lot of traffic should be vacuumed at least once or twice a week. Keep the house free of dust and allergens. Invest in a purifier if possible. Show children by example cleanliness is next to godliness. Children should not be allowed to eat in their bedrooms and all over the house. There should be a designated place for dining.

Plants are great for their energy, beauty, and oxygenation. Flowing water brings a nice calming element to the house; invest in a water fountain or make your own. The home should compliment your child's energy or chi. The kitchen should be a healing and holistic place. It should be kept as clean as possible. The microwave should not be a part of the kitchen. It radiates and kills food, which can lead to cancer. Just being in the presence of microwave can cause various adverse affects: imbalance in hormones, brainwave disturbance, breakdown of human life energy fields, breakdown of cellular brain productions, nervous and lymphatic system damage, changes in intellect, memory loss, stomach and intestinal growth of cancerous tumors and obstructions, and a gradual breakdown of the function of the digestive system.[1] The better organized the kitchen the easier it is to accomplish tasks. Designate a spot for healing herbs. Place them in dark glass jars to keep them fresh. Appliances such as blenders, food processors, and juicers cut down on food prep time. Use stainless steel and cast–iron pots. Do not use aluminum pots. The aluminum can leach into food.

House plants not only beautify the home, but purify the air. Some of the best plant purifiers are the Chinese evergreen, spider plant, golden pothos, peace lily, rubber plant, and Boston fern. Some plants are toxic and poisonous. Keep these plants out of reach or out of the home. Research all plants before bringing them into the home.

Be mindful of the colors you paint your house. Kitchens are usually hot, so choose colors that are cooling. Some prefer greens because they are healing. The kitchen is a place for creating healing foods. Bedrooms are a restful place, so you may want to have calming colors like shades of blue. The living room should be a warm room with inviting colors.

Diodes

The family's electromagnetic fields must be protected. Many man-made electronic devices also have an electronic magnetic field. These especially can be harmful to humans. Today, many experience EMF pollution. The symptoms can be stress, fatigue, headaches, etc. Some EMFs can also cause cancer. If the fields of humans are not harmonious with the fields of man-made electronic devices they can be poisoned by them. A good method of protection is to use neutralizing devices such as diodes. Diodes manage the flow of electrical currents providing balance. The diodes balance energy fields. Diodes can protect the body and its organs from harmful radiation. Humans are exposed to EMF radiation via television, cell phones, computers, and kitchen appliances. The cell phone EMFs are especially dangerous because they are placed directly on the head. Diodes can protect families from EMFs. The insides of homes are electrically wired. The outside has electrical towers and lines. It is essential that usage of electronic devices in the home be limited. The family's television time should be limited also. Diodes are essential when watching television or using the DVD player. The resting place should have as little electrical devices as possible. Limiting the bedroom's electrical devices to just a lamp and clock or less would be ideal. Alarms should not be kept close to the head. Make use of daylight in the home. Limit artificial light. In your work environment ask if the fluorescent lights directly over your head can be removed. This will help reduce much stress and tension. I had maintenance remove them for me at my place of work. I felt better instantly. Many diodes can be attached onto devices or placed under them. They can be carried in pockets and crystal diode jewelry can be worn. The herb white chrysanthemum is another option for protection against radiation. It is also a great detoxifier. White chrysanthemum makes a delicious tea.

Natural Home Cleaning and Pest Control

There are many reasons to consider using natural cleaning and pest control products. The chemicals in them are harsh on the earth and the human body. These chemicals affect pregnant mothers and unborn babies, as well as the health of the family. Not only are these products toxic, but dangerous if a child is to get their hands on them and ingest orally. Do not use plates and utensils cleaned with toxins. Nor, wash your clothes with chemicals that will touch the skin, which can enter the bloodstream. Natural cleaners and pest control products can be purchased from health stores or made at home. One of the most universal home cleaning products is vinegar. Keep a spray bottle filled with equal parts water and vinegar. This will work great on dirt, grease, and scum. It can be used on tabletops, tiles, high chairs, glass tables, mirrors, toilets, carpet stains, and more. Adding vinegar to laundry can even soften the clothes. Second on the list is baking soda. It can be used as a scouring powder, deodorizer, and general cleaner. Add a small amount of baking soda in water for a general cleaner. If you are using baking soda for scouring, add it to the surface using a damp rag. For tougher scouring jobs add salt.

Furniture Polish
- 1 cup olive oil (or oil of your choice).
- ½ cup lemon juice.
- A few drops of lemon essential oil are optional.

Cleaning Drains
- ½ cup of baking soda.
- Followed by 1 cup of vinegar.
- Wait 15 minutes and let the hot water run. Repeat if necessary.

Fleas
- Sprinkle boric acid into the carpets and sweep it in.
- Let this sit for 3-5 days and vacuum.
- Rub fennel powder into the coats of the animal to keep fleas off.

Cockroaches
Place boric acid in places where they frequent, such as baseboards and cabinets.

Mice

Place peppermint essential oil in the places where the mice frequent. Mice detest peppermint oil. To keep mice out of your home grow peppermint around the house.

Ants
Place cinnamon in the cracks or crevices where the ants are entering.

Natural Personal Care

Most personal care products contain toxins and dangerous chemicals. Parents should not use them on their skin or their children's skin. The popular commercial brand baby products are toxic, do not be fooled. More than one-third of all personal care products contain at least one ingredient linked to cancer, according to the nonpartisan, nonprofit EWG (Environmental Working Group), while more than three-quarters may contain harmful impurities such as known carcinogens.[2] Ingredients unknown and hard to pronounced should not be used. Plant derived products should be used on the skin, not synthetics. Natural products can be purchased in natural food stores or be made at home. The toxin mineral oil, a by-product of petroleum, should not be used on the skin. It does not moisturize, it clogs pores. The skin can be moisturized with simple oils such as jojoba, olive, and almond oil. Essential oils can be added for its aromatherapy and healing properties. Shea butter from Afrika provides excellent moisture for the skin. Cocoa butter can also be used. Shampoos can be made at home using castile soaps and essential oils. Most commercial shampoos have skin irritants and toxic chemicals. Natural deodorants should also be used. The commercial brands contain toxins and aluminum, as well as other metals that can be absorbed through the skin and enter the blood stream. Aluminum has been linked to Alzheimer's disease.

Natural fluoride-free toothpaste should be used. Fluoride is toxic, it is a poison. Many commercial toothpastes have labels stating to keep out of reach of children. Most children swallow toothpaste, so they are easily exposed. Children who digest large amounts of fluoride can become ill and even die. Fluoride is believed to harden tooth enamel, but also can cause fluorosis, which can

126

weaken teeth. Tooth powders can be made at home to clean teeth with things such as baking soda, ground cinnamon powder, and ground neem powder.

Toys for Children

When I think about my childhood toys, the first thing that comes to mind is my wooden blocks. I also remember musical instruments, a xylophone in particular. I remember these toys so clearly. These were simple toys that provided everlasting memories. My pre-school memories of toys were also wooden. I went to Montessori schools and the toys were very holistic and natural feeling. I can remember playing with a wooden iron and ironing board. The playhouses and the kitchen sets were also wooden. These toys are not seen too much in mainstream toy stores. Children's toys are mainly computerized and plastic.

Play is great for the health of children. But most of the toys children play with are quite unnatural. Basic wooden toys are available which are entertaining and safe. Choose wooden toys free of toxic paint. Toys such as puppet shows, games, puzzles, workbenches, trucks, construction sets, houses, and boats are available. Afrikan children need to play with toys that are imaginative. Most wooden toys are simple and allow the mind more freedom to innovate and create. Most mainstream toys condition the child's mind to think a certain way. Take time out to look at the types of games or toys that left an impression on your spirit as a child.

In some cultures wood is considered an element. Wood can also be looked at as an earth element. It represents planning, organization, and emotional expression. Wood is also connected to the muscles and eyes; you can clearly see how wooden toys are ideal. The people of Mali and Senegal regard wood as sacred, wood is an extension of the earth and is a symbol of protection, stability, and prosperity.[3] The elements of the universe provide divine order for child's play. Another reason to use more wooden toys is the toxins in some plastic toys. Many toys are made of polyvinyl chloride, also known as PVC. Some PVCs contain phthalates. Phthalates are linked to cancer and kidney damage. Phthalates are especially used in soft toys such as teethers. Its makes the PVC soft. Some plastic toys also have chlorine based chemicals. Chlorine creates the toxin dioxin. Chemicals have the ability to be released from the PVC. These chemicals can be ingested by children. Metals such as led and cadium can also be in plastics. Plastics such as polypropylene and polyethylene are safer. Plastic is synthetic. The more natural the lifestyle, the healthier children will be.

The Toxic Black Hair Care Industry Poisoning Children and the Home
Many Afrikan young girls still playing with toys are having dangerous, caustic, and toxic chemicals placed on their heads. This is done in the pursuit to destroy the natural kinky and highly melanated hair of the Afrikan. The chemicals in hair relaxers are harmful to the stylist placing the chemicals in the child's hair, as well as the child. Fumes are released into the home or salon. The child breathes this all in. The chemicals are then placed directly on the skin. These chemicals go well beyond just the skin, but into the bloodstream. This process becomes a ritual of poisoning the environment as well as the child with toxins. Afrikan mothers must encourage natural hair. They should also know how to maintain it. Unfortunately, many women have forgotten. Due to slavery and colonization, many Afrikan women have had chemically processed hair in the past or present. Some parents may have chemically processed their child's hair and may not be sure how to reverse the process. Other parents may have children with natural hair, but are not exactly sure how to properly take care of their child's hair.

Hair relaxers whether marketed as Lye or No-Lye are toxic. Lye relaxers contain Sodium Hydroxide. No-Lye relaxers contain Guanidine Hydroxide. The truth is, they both are lies! There are no natural hair relaxers. The chemical lye is found in oven and drain cleaners. Relaxers have the ability to clean filthy toilet bowls with hard to remove grime many commercial cleaners cannot. These chemicals should not be placed on the heads of children. Hair relaxers are caustic chemicals and are even considered to be hazardous household waste by the Los Angeles County Department of Public Works Environmental Programs Division.[4] Straightening combs are also dangerous. The extreme heat weakens the hair and many children are sometimes burned by the comb.

Afrikan women have been taught their scalps must be greased. However, most grease contains mineral oil (pertroluem/pertrolatum) which is toxic. This ingredient does not moisturize the hair, but does the exact opposite. Shea butter, jojoba oil, and almond oil are a healthier option. Essential oils can also be added to the hair oil of your choosing. Great essential oils for the hair are rosemary, eucalyptus, ylang ylang, lavender, and geranium. Essential oils can irritate the skin and must be diluted. Always use essential oils in an oil base or water.

When shampooing the child's hair use all natural shampoos. Over the counter shampoos found in markets and beauty supply stores have toxic chemicals that can enter the child's bloodstream. Natural shampoos and conditioners can be found in health food stores. Ingredients such as propylene glycol are found in shampoos. This is the main ingredient in brake fluid and anti-freeze. Sodium lauryl sulfate (SLS) found in most shampoos, is sometimes a skin irritant. Formaldehyde is also in shampoos, including the most popular baby shampoos. The ingredient commonly found in shampoos is Quaternium-15. It is a preservative that releases formaldehyde. Formaldehyde is very toxic and may cause cancer. Many hair products including conditioners marketed towards Afrikan children contain hormones and estrogen that causes early puberty.

Styling Tips

Cherie King, author of *Her Special Hair: A Guide to Understanding & Caring for Your Biracial or African American Daughters Highly Textured Hair*, recommends detangling thick, long hair in sections and then loosely twisting the hair before washing. Part the hair into sections. Use a wide tooth comb starting at the ends and work your way to the root. After detangling each section place the hair into twist. Next, shampoo the hair with the twist still in the hair. Work your way from the scalp to the ends. If the child's hair still has the twists after washing and conditioning. Unravel one twist. Detangle and moisturize, and either twist or plait the hair. Do the same for the rest of the twist. If the twists unravel after washing, section the hair again, detangle, moisturize, and add plaits or twist. This will set the hair. Setting the hair provides manageability for styling the hair the next day. The hair can be styled while wet for plaits, cornrows or two-strand twists. Blow drying the hair is an option, but can cause breakage. Blow dry the child's hair in moderation.

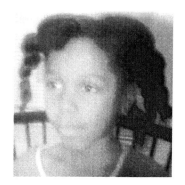 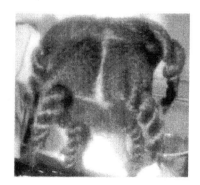

Courtesy of Cherie King

Relaxers can be cut out of the hair. They can be removed slowly by cutting the relaxed ends by what is called transitioning. The child's hair can be kept in styles such, as braids, cornrows, pony tails, and two-strand twist. Avoid heat when transitioning and keep the hair well moisturized. Cherie King recommends cutting off 1-3 inches of hair every couple of months or so. When the hair is at a comfortable length for parents and the child all the remaining ends can be cut off.

Picture of a transition style

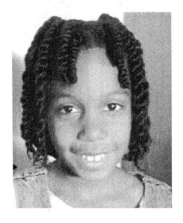

Courtesy of Cherie King

Pictures of natural hair styles

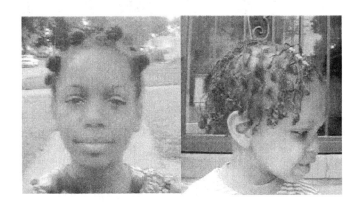

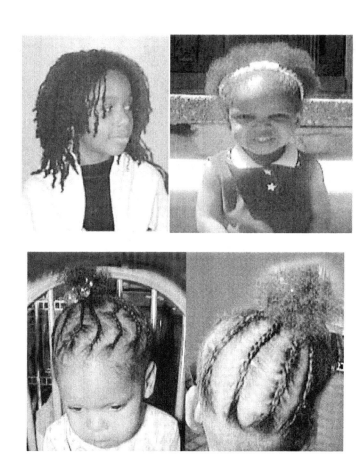

Pictures Courtesy of Cherie King

Afrikan children's natural hair is beautiful. Harmful chemicals which hurt their bodies and minds are not needed. Mothers must lead by example, wearing regal crowns which are chemical and toxic free. Lead the way, be a shining example of what an Afrikan woman is and should be.

Television and Music
Television programming does just that, program. It has the ability to program children's thought processes. If parents choose to allow their children to watch television, the program should be age appropriate and not psychologically and spiritually damaging. The time watched should also be limited. Play time should be exploring nature, creating, and loving. Not spending the majority of time in front of an object that is emitting radiation. Children's mental and physical health should be protected. Viktoras Kulvinskas, author of the book *Survival into the 21ˢᵗ Century* describes television:

> Of all synthetic pacifiers, television is probably the most pernicious, instrumental in spiritual, mental, and physical deterioration of the growing child. Materialistic commercials equate love with food, possessions, and sensuality. Children are bombarded with details of violence, drugs, drunkenness, and war. All too often this view becomes the children's real world, distorting even forming, their values and separating them from emotional involvement with people, creating a perverted view of God and nature.[5]

The majority of the commercials on television are not Afrikan centered. Much of it is of no use to Afrikan families. The programs available consist of buffoonery, booty shaking, violence, and sex. The only images shown of the Afrikan continent are of war and poverty. DVDs are a better option if parents choose to have a television in the home at all. Parents should watch DVDs first before allowing their children to view them. The movie *Kirikou and the Sorceress* is a DVD about an Afrikan child and his village. It is Afrikan and family oriented. Choose cultural films rich in history.

Radio stations also program. Music carries vibrations that affect the chakra system. Music is very magical. Music is a tool through which the artist has the ability to pass their emotions on to the listener. Children do not know how to detach, some adults do not. Allow children to listen to uplifting music, like Bob Marley for example. Let them listen to chants of liberation. Program liberation into the child's spirit. Instrumental music will allow children to lay their own emotions on the music. This way they can transfer their emotions to music and filter it properly instead of others transferring their thoughts onto the child. The music being marketed towards Afrikan children is being used as a tool to keep them asleep and participants in degenerate behavior. Many of the popular music artists are pedophiles, violent, abusive towards women, and uneducated. The music promotes gross capitalism that puts money in every community, but Afrikan communities. Children must understand that if this behavior continues they will be a permanent underclass in America. Afrikans are running out of time and have no place for music in their lives that does not uplift, educate, and create a sense of pride, love, and divinity. The best music for children to listen to is the music they actually created. Invest in instruments for children.

Family Rituals

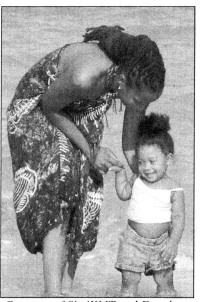

Courtesy of Sha'KMT and Freedom,
Photography by Baba Born Divine

Family time is essential. Rituals can be centered around creating music, singing, playing board games, story telling, dancing, yoga, travel, eating, and star gazing. The only ritual many Afrikan

134

children today partake in, is television. The television is how children spend their leisure time. The ancestors were great astronomers, architects, healers, story tellers, and artists because they had leisure time. However, they used their time wisely and television did not occupy the homes to divert their attention to an object that causes the brain to flat line. Many parents spend most of their leisure time with their children in front of the television. Television does not promote creativity or strengthen family bonds. Children need quality and productive family time.

Dinner time is the easiest and best time for the family to sit together and bond. Children need to see the family breaking bread together. This time should be healing physically, mentally, and spiritually. Make it a sacred event held in a designated clean and peaceful space.

I once was watching a sistren's children. I thought they needed to calm down, so I taught them yoga. They enjoyed doing the many postures, meditating, and finding a quiet place within themselves. When I taught them yoga I had no idea the impact that it would leave on them. I never told their mother that we did yoga. Their mother later told me the children were doing yoga and meditating. Children want to do so much more than play with toys, video games, and watch television. Children want to have interaction with their elders and parents. Families should take time out to participate in rituals based on family fun. Play board games as a family; parents will be surprised how much children enjoy these games once introduced. Sing and dance with your children. Invest in instruments, so they can actually provide the music to sing and dance too. Storytelling is such an important part of the Afrikan oral tradition. Keep this tradition alive by passing these stories down to the next generation. Star gazing is also a great activity many Afrikan children have no exposure too. Invest in a telescope if you have the funds. The ancestors charted the stars without the help of the modern technology we have today. Children need to see our universe, not just the earth. Educate the children and have fun at the same time. There are a multitude of ways families can bond and grow. Be creative and simply let the divine inspire your family to create your own sacred rituals.

Building Healthy Communities

Parenthood is easier with support from extended family members and friends. Help allows mothers and fathers to attend business, do chores, and have leisure time. Parenthood can become exhausting without some extra help now and then. Some parents do not live close to relatives, so it is imperative networks are built, so communities can be created for children. Like-minded holistic parents need to build support groups. New mothers especially, need free time to take a shower or make a meal. Some mothers just want to enjoy a meal. Mothers appreciate it when a sista friend can come by and help out for the day. Not only is she getting help around the house, but also feminine adult company and energy in the home. It may not seem like much, but mothers appreciate it. Many mothers do not feel comfortable leaving their children with others who do not have the same value systems. Sistren can baby-sit for other mothers, bringing the importance of community back into the Afrikan culture again.

The community can preserve traditions while improving the quality of life of families. Some parents work and go to school and cannot always afford or want their children in daycare. So, it is up to the community to build strong networks. Sista circles and tea party type events allow networking that will provide mothers with emotional, spiritual, and physical support. Women can share ideas and entrepreneurial pursuits. Bonds and friendships can be formed that will allow sistren to have physical support such as baby-sitting. It is imperative the community take responsibility for all the children.

Children need love and support. In traditional Afrikan villages, children are allowed to spend time in the homes of the community. Mothers and fathers do not stress when a child cannot be found in the home. Parents know their children are being well taken care of. Children are the blessings of the community. Therefore, Afrikans must form networks that create a space that will allow them to flourish and fulfill their purpose on their journey. Children have chosen to bless the community, return the blessing.

Alternative Energy for Afrikans
An interview with Bro. Levi Hoodari SunguRa, of The Institute of Urban Survival Science & Technology.

How can solar energy benefit Afrikans living in urban communities?
The energy system chosen should be in accordance with the environment and the seasons. If I am in a rural environment where there is plenty of sunlight, the amount of heat that I would receive makes it easier to do things such as solar water heating. A light water absorber, a panel that absorbs sunlight and heats up the piping and tubing for the water can be used. This can be done in a nice rural environment. In places such as the city, where urbanized Afrikans reside during the harsher seasons hot water may not heat up as well.

The system used in the city would be electric solar panels connected to a battery system, amplified by an inverter and directed through the house. Recently, in my studies I have found that you can use 48–60 volts DC of electricity. The heat in the house can run off a 12-24 volts DC power supply connected to an inverter. The inverter multiplies the electricity to 120 or 240 volts AC. This method allows the heater to be used. If you live in a two level house, one heater can be placed on the first floor, blowing heat currents through the home. The second can be placed in the hallways on the floor.

The next appliance is an electric hot water heater. This requires another 12-24 volts DC. A 12 volt power supply is connected to an inverter connected to an electrical water heater. This can be accomplished with 12–24 volts DC according to the type of system you design.

Solar energy can also be used for the stove. Families would need to have an electric stove. The stove can also run off a 12-24 volt DC power supply hooked up to an inverter. This will amplify the 12-24 DC volts and give them 120-240 AC volts.

In regards to lighting, it can all be run with a small amount of voltage with high output. You can have a 3 volt, 6 volt, or 9 volt light in the front room, kitchen, hallways, and the bedrooms. The batteries are constantly being recharged by sunlight.

If still hooked up to the grid you can sell electricity back to the electric company. Electricity goes back through the wires of your house. This causes the electric meter to reverse. You are now sending electricity out. The electricity can be sold back to the electric company giving you a discount.

When dealing with major electrical appliances everything can run with 12-24 volts DC. Each battery and inverter is being recharged by solar panels. The only thing that differs is the amount of sunlight familes get during the seasons. So, during harsh seasons especially, conserve energy. When the lights do not need to be used keep them off. Use daylight instead. As far as the heating is concerned, make sure the cracks in the walls and windows are sealed properly. Windows sealed properly or caulked saves energy. Place towels at the bottom of front doors. Insulate the house, so heat is not escaping. Proper insulation and proper use of light is essential. Use the stove only when needed. Hot water can be conserved too.

An initial 12 volts DC each for the stove, hot water, heater, and lights are needed. That is basically 36-72 volts of electricity all managed by you. There is nothing to pay. Once it is built, it is built. You only have to deal with maintenance.

What is the start up cost?
It varies depending on where familes get their equipment from. If they purchase heavy duty solar panels it can cost anywhere from $200-$1000. If they go with a smaller system, a small panel can cost $20-$100. It is also according to how many things familes are running to determine how many solar panels they need. Inverters can cost $10. One inverter is needed for each system or appliance.

What is a good appliance if someone wants to start out small and just see how solar energy works?
Families can start off with the lights. The lights are something you can plug in because the inverter has an outlet plug. For that

outlet plug they can get voltage dividers. With these dividers families can run lamps. A 3 volt lamp in each room can illuminate the whole room. The next easiest is the stove. Families must first have an electric stove. Most stoves require 240 volts. They will also need an inverter.

I will explain the inverter. The inverter is a small apparatus. It is a voltage amplifier. It amplifies DC volts and converts it to AC voltage. AC is alternating current which is used for most appliances. You can amplify 24-240 volts AC and run an electric stove off of it.

Is solar energy more ideal for warm places such as Afrika or the Caribbean?
It is most definitely ideal. It is perfect for those areas. For the urban area it is perfect also. But, for the urban area, it is best to have it integrated with batteries and small generator systems for back up. If still hooked up to the grid, the batteries can be re-charged off of it. However, most likely if you are preserving your energy, have a tight design, or tight structure you will not have to recharge your battery much from an outside source. You can integrate your system by having small generators. Periodically recharge the battery with your generator. Families can also have a stand by re-charger, a car battery charger that stays plugged in to a source. So, when the battery starts to go weak around the cellar basement or chamber they know that each battery is getting 30 minutes of juice and to recharge your battery.

Can more be done in rural warm climates?
Yes, families can do a lot more in rural warm areas. They can have more than solar energy. Wind energy is available too. Families can work off the grid or use gas. Biomass can be used if close to a farm. Biomass is organic materials. It can be burned creating all types of oils from the animals around. Biomass can be used to make methane gas. Warm areas are beautiful for alternative energy.

Do you think rural areas are more ideal for Afrikans to be self – sufficient?

It would be more appreciable and beneficial if we were in a more rural area or society. The advantage of the city is being closer to commerce. You are constantly getting electrical appliances coming in and out the city. Families can create or upgrade their system more easily. The benefit of a rural society is having more systems available. Families can catch energy from the sun, wind, tides in the earth, and waste material. They don't have to worry about generators bothering neighbors. But, there are cases for generators to muffle the sound.

Can everyday people learn to use alternative energy? Is a science background needed?
Families do not have to have a long science background. But, they have to have a good comprehension of how things work, knowing how to put things together, and following instructions. Families must have a basic understanding of environment. An everyday person can have good electrical heater or space fan that can run off of 12 volts DC of electricity, blowing hot air through the house. An average person can run and create that. It is not hard to manage or maintain.

Were you good in math and science in high school?

I studied Science as a hobby in high school. It was when I went to college that I took environmental science.

Why do you think Afrikan children shy away from Science and math?
It is the way we are being taught. Our education is being shown from a standpoint of training and not life. We are not experiencing our learning. People speak about science as if it is separate from everyday life. We are being taught from an external non-intimate process. This is being done on purpose to create a serving class. Our grandparents, people in the late 19th century and early 20th centuries created the best inventions with the least amount of education. This is because the early education was learning through doing. Education was hands on and integrated. Black children do not learn like this today. It is two dimensional learning in a three dimensional world. In the past it was learning how to use tools and learning how to do experiments. Children

now only learn on paper. Our grandparents learned through using tools. It is the way we are being taught.

Is alternative energy a must for Afrikans?
Yes.
1. Self-Sufficiency. If you control the energy of your society, you can control the prosperity and production of the people. You can dictate the rate at which that society excels.
2. With the current energy crisis it is most felt by the poorer people with price hikes and taxes.
3. Control, you are able to supply energy and maintain a home environment that is not risking the health of children or industry. You are protecting your children.

7 - Education

Infant and Toddler Development

The child's education begins in the womb. Parents must be mindful of their thoughts and interactions with others. The unborn child is learning in the womb. The child hears the words and feels the emotions of the outside world. If parents wish for their children to be musical geniuses they should expose their unborn to music such as the jazz of John Coltrane, Thelonius Monk, Sun Ra, and Charles Mingus. Let the child hear the dynamic drumming of Baba Olatunji. Recite mathematical equations and read to the unborn. Be mindful that if there is chaos and negativity in your environment the baby will learn this too. The type of primordial education the unborn receives is the parent's choice.

It is never too early to begin educating infants and toddlers. Babies need interaction and stimulus. Parents should look their babies in the eyes, smile, and talk to them. Parents who do things such as, explain the body parts and talk to their children while getting them dressed, will have children who begin communicating much earlier. Children especially need loving parents. When performing tasks around the home, parents should tell their children what they are doing. Make them feel included. While I am cooking, I give my son a pot and spoon allowing him to cook too. He sometimes tells me he wants to eat. I explain to him I am cooking and he understands to wait patiently. He is only twenty-three-months-old, but understands his food will be coming soon. Encourage their language skills. Help children to speak the words they wish to communicate. Proper communication eliminates a lot of negative behavior. Children get upset and engage in activities which parents disapprove of when they are bored or ignored. They want to learn. Children are going to want to explore the home and touch things. Let them do it. Make the home appropriate for children. A designated play area is a good for keeping the rest of the home tidy. Play is education for children. Parents should play with them. As stated in an earlier chapter, basic wooden toys that allow imagination are great for children. Simple stacking blocks, puzzles, and activity boxes are great. Play, such as, putting clothes in the laundry basket and doing chores around the house are great fun for children. Provide activities that encourage problem solving, but be very aware not to push them beyond their level of development. Reading is especially important. It is fun for children and their parents, enhancing the child's communication skills. The book *Awakening the Natural Genius of Black Children* states:

> The child who does well has a mother or caregiver who provides a rich variety of objects and toys for play allows freedom to roam and discover, gives attention to her child when he finds something unusually exciting or when he encounters something difficult to overcome, turns everyday situations into games and talks to her child.[1]

The Afrikan child has so much potential to excel educationally. However, in the Diaspora the Afrikan child continues to lag behind educationally. Afrikan children are born with above average sensorimotor and brain power. Marcelle Geber's 1958 study and research of Ugandan children testifies to the advance motor skills of Afrikan children:

> She [Marcelle Geber] used the famous Gesell tests for early intelligence, developed at Yale University's child development center. The pictures of the forty-eight-hour-old child-supported only by the forearms, bolt, upright perfect head balance and eye focus, and a marvelous intelligence shinning in the face- are no more astonishing than those of the six-week - old child. At six or seven weeks...these children crawled skillfully, could sit spellbound before a mirror looking at their images for long periods. This particular ability was not expected in the American-European child before twenty-four weeks (six months) according to the Gesell tests. Between six and seven months, the Uganda children performed the toy-box retrieval tests. Geber showed the infant a toy, walked across the room, put the toy in a tall toy box; the child leaped up, ran across the room, and retrieved the toy.[1]

The Kikuyu children of Kenya were also studied in 1973 by Leiderman and associates in accordance with the Bayley scales of infant development. The Bayley scales measure physical and mental functions. During the fifteen months of testing Kikuyu children outscored Black and White children in the United States

143

and United Kingdom. Afrikans all over the world have the intellectual ability to control the Afrikan continent and resources. But, on the continent Afrikans are not controlling their resources. Colonization has ended, but the resources are still controlled by the "ex"colonizers. In America, Afrikans do not operate the majority of businesses in their neighborhoods, nor do they govern themselves. There is no reason why this reality has to remain when Afrikan children have such bright minds. The minds of children in America are cultivated by the media and teachers that are largely White females. This type of education will not allow Afrikan children to have the drive or the ability to control resources, community, and family. It is no coincidence that many Afrikan leaders on the Afrikan continent who mismanage their governments were educated in either the United States or Europe. Parents must support the Afrikan child's abilities and provide the proper tools for intellectual superiority. The Afrikans removal from traditional Afrikan society has created dysfunctional families. Afrikans now either have an American dream or no dream at all. This dream or lack or dream molds the way children are raised and educated. In traditional Afrikan society parenthood is only allowed after rites of passage. Marriage and childbearing were permitted only after completion of training and initiation. In this way, the parents and adults who reared children, did so on the basis of an accordance with consistent, shared values, perspectives, and social goals.[1] Afrikan children of the Diaspora are not being educated or raised to meet social goals.

Afrikan–Centered Independent Schools and Homeschooling

Education must provide a means of social advancement for the Afrikan community. Education should not be a piece paper that makes a graduate proud to hold. Education should make Afrikans proud to own black-owned businesses, maintain two-parent homes, engage in global trade, and govern their own communities. The public and private schools that are not Afrikan centered will not give the Afrikan child the tools to build the Afrikan community or home. They will receive a mentality to work for the advancement of other cultures or a do-for-self mentality. Some parents may see nothing wrong with this. They are happy their children are being educated to get a job. Dr. Amos Wilson pointed out in one of his lectures about Afrikan males being placed in special education class that Afrikans do not have the same problems as Caucasians. They have different social, political, and economical issues. How can a white female teacher teach Afrikan children to become socially, economically, and politically empowered? The American system disempowers Afrikan children and empowers the Caucasian. They cannot and will not teach Afrikan children to become empowered. The children will be taught to keep working for the system which is disenfranchising them, instead of revolting against the system. Children learn early in school not to demand change from the American government or school system. Everyday when they go to school, they pledge allegiance to the American flag. Many children are not taking the time out each day to pledge allegiance to their spirit, ancestors, communities, or families. This is one of the reasons why children do not value their communities. They have not been taught to have an allegiance to Afrikan values. In Nah Dove's book *Afrikan Mothers Bearers of Culture and Social Change* she asserts:

> They must have an allegiance to Afrikan people predicated upon a vision of the future outside that conceived by the oppressor. Afrikan mothers and fathers who send their children to culturally affirming schools have begun the process for their children because generally they are aware of the distinctions between schooling for subjugation and education for liberation.[2]

The Marcus Garvey School founded by Dr. Palmer in 1979 is one of the best Afrikan–centered schools in the United States. The school is for grades pre–school through eighth-grade. The achievements of the Marcus Garvey School are exceptional:

> Two-year-olds learn to recite their alphabets in English, Swahili, and Spanish. Three-year-olds can recite the Latin names of all the major bones in the body and can recognize all fifty states on the map, can name all the states and cite their capitals with the minimal assistance of their teachers. It is a commonplace for four-year-old preschoolers to read from third through sixth grade books...At Garvey, algebra is taught in the fourth grade and trigonometry and calculus taught in the early grades. Garvey third grade students scored higher on both reading and math than sixth graders from a public school for gifted

(predominately White children) on identical tests administered to both classes.[1]

Accredited independent Afrikan schools are becoming popular in the United States, United Kingdom, and Canada. These schools give children a sense of pride, knowledge of self, and the ability to learn in an environment especially designed for their advancement. Some schools provide vegetarian lunches. High sugar foods such as candy and soda are prohibited to ensure the child's diet does not interfere with their leaning. The Afrikan independent school liberates the Afrikan child through education. No oppressor is going to design a curriculum which puts the whip in the oppressee's hands. Afrikans do not need equal education, but better education. Many Afrikan children in so-called "third world" countries have fewer supplies, and the school structures are sometimes dilapidated. However, these children are more advanced than the United States' inner city children. Some countries have an Afrikan teacher dedicated to their education. Before the civil rights era many Afrikan children were excelling in segregated schools. The schools were then integrated creating a brain drain. Afrikan children are not encouraged to be employers, but employees in the integrated schools. Nor, are these schools centers for the advancement of the community's spiritual, social, and economical progress. Afrikans in the United States are consumers not producers. They do not need to go to school to learn how to get a job and simply consume. Afrikans need schools that teach them how to become producers and create jobs.

Home schooling and Afrikan–centered schools are the best options for Afrikan boys and girls. If these two alternatives to the traditional school system are not available to parents another option is Afrikan-centered Saturday schools. These schools can be run by the community on a volunteer basis. Community is vital if Afrikans are to begin educating their children for liberation. Stay-at-home parents can open their homes to children of parents who cannot provide home schooling. Traditional schooling can be damaging to Afrikan children and should be avoided if possible. It is especially damaging to Afrikan boys. They live in a patriarchal society where men are expected to be aggressive and women submissive. This is an issue for Afrikan boys because they are feared by White society, and any sign of aggression adds to this fear. The majority of teachers are White females. Many White females have a natural fear of Afrikan males. Girls have fewer issues because they take more submissive roles in schools. Because of this, Afrikan girls are less targeted in the American school system and are not quick to be labeled as students with special needs or behavioral problems. Boys are being labeled as young as kindergarten. Jawanza Kunjufu in his book *Countering The Conspiracy to Destroy Black Boys* states:

> How much academic information do teachers have on a child on the eighth day of kindergarten? They have very little. They rely on the social worker's interview and the parental registration forms. They also take a look at how children are dressed, the way the smell, whether they are verbal with adults, whether they speak Black English, whether the father is in the home, whether they're low income and what their energy level is in the classroom. Children who do not meet the teacher's feminine, middle-class standard are placed in the lowest reading group.[3]

Many teachers label Afrikan boys as slow and place them in remedial classes because they appear slower compared to Afrikan girls. Girls mature two years ahead of boys, so it appears the boys are slower. The boys do not have issues learning, boys and girls simply learn differently. This difference is not a reason to label boys as needing special education, but many teachers are doing just that. Jawanza Kunjufu also suggests an all Black male classroom taught by a Black male, so there would not be a need for comparisons. Afrikan boys are disportionately placed in special education compared to Afrikan girls and Caucasian boys and girls. They do not have problems learning, just problems learning in the traditional school system. Afrikans cannot expect programs such as "No child left behind" to save their children. The community must step up and take control of their children's education. Many parents are taking control; Afrikans are the fastest growing segment of home schoolers.

Schools that are earth friendly also add to the child's well - being. Some schools are now being built that have solar panels, photovoltaic cells on roof tops, ice plants for air conditioning, recycled flooring, and roof–top water conservation for toilet

147

flushing. New York State requires schools to use green cleaners. Pesticides are also being curbed in some schools. Natural methods are being used to rid the schools of pest, preventing exposure to toxins, carcinogens, and chemicals that cause neurological damage. Earth friendly schools are using low-VOC (Volatile Organic Compounds) paints, adhesives, and sealants during construction. Daylight is being used more than fluorescent light, saving energy. Daylight helps students achieve higher test scores. The article "great green schools" published by *Mothering* magazine states:

> In a 1999 study conducted in Seattle, Washington, and Fort Collins, Colorado, students in classes with the most daylight were found to have higher test scores than those in classes with the least daylighting. More dramatic results were found in a school in Capistrano, California, where, in one year, classes with the most daylight progressed 20 percent faster on reading test than those with the least daylight.[4]

Schools that take a holistic approach to the environment produce brighter children. Diet is being emphasized in some schools. Organic gardening and healthier cooking are being taught. Healthy diet contributes to better behavior, development, and learning. Schools without chemical irritants and allergens are preventing asthma attacks, headaches, and other ailments, because the air is cleaner.

Homeschooling provides children with a curriculum, Afrikan and family centered. Parents do not have to worry about de-programming their children when they return home from school. The child's diet does not have to be compromised in school. Most schools only have unhealthy food available and many children share food. Homeschooling can put the parent's mind at ease because they are in total control of their child's education. It usually requires one parent to stay at home or work part-time. Teenage children do much of their learning on their own, so homeschooling does not require as much time of the parents. Critics will argue homeschooling will cause the child to be less social. Children can have after school and weekend activities with other children. Playmates are also available in the neighborhood. Parents must also ask themselves if the socialization their children

148

are experiencing in public schools is healthy. Children who want to actually learn in school are sometimes harassed. Numerous fights take place in the schools. Many of the children are unruly and prevent other children from learning. Children can learn dysfunctional social behaviors in traditional schools. Behaviors parents did not send their child to school with. Afrikan male youth are especially suffering in traditional schools.

Homeschooling is legal. The right of parents to homeschool their children was first established in 1974 in a New Mexico Supreme Court case.[5] Parents do not need to have teaching experience or be certified to teach. Afrikan centered e-learning is available through the Aya Educational Institute (http://www.ayaed.com). Parents and children can take interactive classes online. Some classes include advanced mathematics, Afrikan history, and science courses. Afrikan languages such as Twi and Yoruba are taught. Serious books are studied such as Amos Wilson's *The Blueprint to Black Power* and *Falsification of African Consciousness*. SAT Prep is also offered. Afrikan parents do have resources. Homeschooling is becoming easier than ever.

Homeschooled children can attend college. Although most colleges and universities ask for high school transcripts or a diploma in their applications, homeschoolers have been successful at getting into college without either. Most colleges require homeschoolers to take the Scholastic Aptitude Test (SAT) or American College Test (ACT) for admission.[5]

Afrikan Schooling
By Sa Mut Herr

My experience involving children in schooling with Afrikan heritage has been reassuring and dignified. There is a fulfilling feeling that comes from knowing children are being educated about their roots and acknowledging that they are essentially Afrikan. The first step I made towards involving the children in Afrikan schooling was when I chose to put them in a Kamitic (Ancient Egyptian) cultural home school called Sen Ntui Baa. My son Seshem loved it since he had a close circle of friends in an Afrocentric setting. He learned about Afrikan culture and was

149

taught holistically. He was taught according to where he was at developmentally, without the expectations of where others thought he should be. Not to mention, he was highly supported and nurtured by the other students of the school. What I observed during Seshem's attendance reflected the true and sincere way to school children from an Afrocentric approach.

Some months later, I was contemplating what to do with my children educationally. Since, I did not want the children to attend public school, I thought the best alternative was for me to home school them myself. However, the reality of me needing to work at that time didn't completely support it. So, I decided to take a leap into the unknown and ask a close friend to home school my children. Why? Well I acknowledged his passion for collecting home school material and resources and being highly involved in the community, let alone him being highly involved in his daughter's learning. Therefore, we started a home school with my two children and his daughter in my home. It was a liberating experience. We had the freedom to design and implement our own programs for the children. After a little while the word spread around about our home school. Eventually, more parents decided to bring their children. We soon had a community home school of five children. After a series of events and experiences due to the circumstances at the time, the school ended. In hindsight the children learned to embrace their roots through education. It was definitely memorable, the opportunity to experience schooling on that level.

Sa Mut Herr is a mother of two, yoga instructor, and a Pan-Afrikan networking business owner.

Home Schooling's the Way
By Sherose

Public school ain't free and Private is a fancy name
I've tried both, NOW i'm home schooling
Public put my child to shame, YOU'RE the boss, so whose to blame
Private stole my money, hell, I got sick of their fooling

150

It's all about Race and Money, that School House game
Haven't you heard, they don't TEACH anymore these days
They get paid to tell lies, talk American Idol, fortune and fame
They suck life out of little Black kids, hurt their brains, teach THEIR ways

Public school cost fortunes and you really can't afford to pay
Special Ed Black kids, lost souls, low self-esteem, sexual addicts and more
Private's the same, less students, no difference, PAYING is their way
If you truly love your children you'll eat this apple and see its core

I tell you Teachers don't TEACH no more
They put a book in their hands and a screen to their face
Walk out the room and close the door
Haven't you heard? The program your child's under is called,...Pace

The curriculum of THIS school day?????
Cheerleading for the white girls and sports for the boys
Preselected since first grade and whatever they DO or SAY is the way
The JOYS of school, ALL for THEM and they get all the toys

Homeschooling ain't hard at all, just requires a little of your time
With a highschool diploma you could do it yourself
Or find the home schools on line and pay as you go, a grand and a dime
Look, the schools have failed our children and they need our help

If the Internet Highway is what they're using THERE
Then they can achieve the same results sitting somewhere else
Teacher places a disc in the CD drive with another one to spare
I'm not TOO dumb and they're full of hogwash

In homeschooling they're a few perks too
Fewer school clothes to buy, no gang fights or discriminations to bear
No discussions with teachers who don't have a clue

And you won't have to buy that Air Jordan shoe

Now some may ask, "what about socialization"
You have family and friends, museums and zoos, attend church,
get along with others?
Today's school don't TEACH, they're only for rehabilitation
To destroy the good works of the fathers, tear down the spirit-
filled mothers
They're destroying our children cause Lynch is still living!
Kill Bill??? HELL NO! Kill Willie!!!
Snatch your child! Take some courage! Put your money in one
pot, start a ring!
Remember, Willie has a girlfriend teaching today and her name is
miss White, Lily White

Sherose ©2006

Rites of Passage

Many people will never reach adulthood. Some will be forty-
years-of-age and still be a child. Today's society looks toward the
college universities to prepare young men and women for
adulthood and self-sufficiency. College cannot teach Afrikan men
and women to be accountable for the Afrikan family, community,
and future. Children think that simply reaching a certain age
entitles them to be treated like an adult. Many feel adult behavior
is staying outside the home at late hours, consumerism, and dating.
These are things many so-called adults do long into their lives.
They go to work everyday and spend their money and time on
nonsense. Young Afrikans need training that will prepare them to
be self-sufficient and enrich their communities. They must have
knowledge of self. Roles and responsibilities must be clearly
defined. Afrikans have been winging it for too long, hoping the
children will eventually just grow up and become responsible
adults. In traditional Afrikan societies the whole community is
vested in its children's journey into adulthood. The community
celebrates the youth's progression each step of the way. The
rituals successfully completed are also accomplishments of the
entire community. The initiates are expected to follow the moral

codes they have learned after initiation when they are released back into the community.

Rites of Passage programs can be formed by individuals or the community. Programs can be done in small groups or with just one child.

Suggestions for Rites of Passage Programs

Separation
- Children wear cultural clothes for a period of time removing them from mainstream society.

Understanding Nature
- Children are taught to rely on and respect nature. They learn to grow plants, flowers, and food. A society cannot be self-reliant if they cannot feed themselves. Many urban communities have vacant lots that can be used.
- The importance of conservation is taught.
- Children participate in alternative energy experiments.

Economics
- Children learn banking.
- Identify businesses which the Afrikan community needs.
- Visit Afrikan-owned businesses.
- Learn how to buy wholesale and sell goods.
- Shop only Afrikan or mostly Afrikan. After the end of the exercise, children should have created an Afrikan business directory.

Heal Thyself
- Children are taught about nutrition (children abstain from certain toxic foods such as candy, soda, artificial colors, and preservatives).
- Herbalism (if possible take children on herbal walks to learn how to gather fresh herbs).
- Alternatives views concerning healing and disease.

Afrikan History and Culture

153

- Extensive classes on Afrikan history including reading, videos, museums, and field trips.
- Children attend Afrikan drumming and dance classes.
- Afrikan martial arts such as capoeira can be studied. Contact some of the capoeirista in your community for assistance. If a parent is creating a rites of passage program for their child only, they can enroll the child in a class.
- Children learn Afrikan languages such as Yoruba or Twi. Many Yoruban and Akan communities have classes. The rites of passage directors may be able to use them as a resource.
- Trips to the Afrikan continent can be planned.
- Children communicate with continental Afrikan pen pals.
- At the end of the exercise children should be able to present the benefits of working relationships between continental and diasporic Afrikans working together for economic and social progress. Along with having knowledge and pride of Afrikan culture.

Household
- Children learn to make basic healthy meals.
- Holistic cleaning, benefits of recycling, and maintaining a toxic free home are taught.

Reliability and Cooperation
- Children are given tasks to complete, but all must be done with their partner. This promotes sistahood and brothahood. Children are taught to rely on each other, along with learning how to trust.

Boys Specifically
- Sexuality
- Manhood
- Mate selection
- Fatherhood (Teens who already have children will receive separate training and mentoring).
- Violence Prevention

- Introduction to the trades. Contact carpenters, plumbers, electricians, etc. in the community who might be interested in volunteering.

Girls Specifically
- Sewing
- Crocheting
- Knitting
- Sexuality
- Motherhood (Teens who already have children will receive separate training and mentoring).
- Household maintenance
- Mate selection
- Respecting the body temple (young women can make waist beads they always will keep hidden under their clothes. The waist beads are for young women that have reached fertility. The waist beads are a reminder that no one should see them and to respect her body temple. The beads are only to be seen by the opposite sex upon maturity.
- Girls learn to accept their body types and facial features. Girls who choose to remove chemically treated hair can do so in this exercise and will receive extra kudos. Those who know ahead of time can begin growing their hair out in advance.

The above suggestions are simply ideas. Create a curriculum which is specific to the community's needs.

Conclusion

Afrikans must take back their traditional identity. Most are in limbo, stuck between two worlds. Not alive, nor dead. Conscious children must be birthed. Healing must take place before conception. The community must encourage and guide potential parents. Every child is the community's child and they should be celebrated. The community must look into child's path while they are in the womb. The child's path is the community's path. A community can be going straight, but one child can change its journey. The child can affect the whole. Holistic parenting is needed. Children must be protected from toxic foods, medicine, and environments. Parents should have the authority to parent in their own image. They should feel confident making decisions concerning their child's health, education and well being. Many parents do not have this confidence. They listen to physicians and mainstream society, instead of following their parental instincts.

The future of the Afrikan family is dependent on its children. Many children are out of touch with nature, resulting in a disconnection with themselves. Children can be seen uprooting newly planted trees. They have no problem polluting the land or waters. However, these same children lied in wombs polluted with antibiotics, pesticides, hormones, and fire retardants. Their early beginnings in life were outside of nature. Most hospital birth processes defy nature with over use of medication and hospital tools. After birth many children are bathed and moisturized with toxic body care products. A disposable diaper with toxins is then placed on the baby. This cycle of unnatural lifestyle usually continues throughout the lives of many people up until their deaths. The cycle must be broken through education and action.

The Afrikan child must be raised up onto the shoulders of their parents. There are many things children cannot see. It is the parent's duty to place them in a position where they do have sight. Parents must make success visible. Children must be guided regarding their education, relationships, dreams, and business endeavors. Educationally, the Afrikan male is falling behind. Afrikan relationships are in a state of distress. Some children do not dare to dream. The community does not take the time to encourage children to make their dreams a reality. Instead, children are forced to adapt to the grim reality society has given them. In many communities Afrikan businesses are almost non-existent. A grassroots educational program must be established by the community to address the needs specific to the Afrikan family.

The Afrikan child's physical and mental well-being is being influenced outside of the community and household. Parents must be critical and analyze everything and everyone that comes in contact with their children. Fast food chains are placing replicas of one of the most expensive SUV automobiles in kid's meals. Not only is the child attacked by fast food's hormones, pesticides, antibiotics, gender-bending chemicals, but gross capitalism. Fast food chains are polluting the Afrikan child's body and encouraging them to pollute the land. The bling bling culture has infrutrated the community, especially the poor communities. Children are killing each other to purchase diamonds from an industry that is oppressing the Afrikan family on the continent. The media and other entities encouraging the degeneration of the community must be shut out. The elders are whom the children should be learning from. They should be at the feet of the elders. Children should be eating at the elder's tables, not fast food restaurants. Children need food for their mind and spirit. Children should enjoy a meal where they see it prepared with love. The food preparer's hands passes on history. Bread should be broken in a holistic environment. At the end of each meal the family should be able to leave with more wisdom. Many families do not eat together. Family leisure time is essential. Leisure time has been replaced with individualized inorganic activity. Children must be exposed to parks and the countryside. They need to feel the grass under their bare feet. The cement disconnects the spirit from the earth energy. Time is needed for re-establishing that connection and promoting healing. Communities should take the children out into the open air to drum, sing, and dance. Children should have the experience of sharing a meal cooked over an open fire, followed by sharing stories, and dreams under the stars. Amusement parks, movies theaters, and malls are not the only outlets for fun times. Inner-city families who have the luxury of traveling should visit rural areas in the Americas, Afrika, and the

157

Caribbean islands, and get away from the concrete. Many parents will see their children's allergies and asthmatic conditions improve. Their spiritual and emotional well-being will also be recharged.

The home should be a place where the children experience a recharge also. It should be a place the children want to come home too. Do not allow the streets to be more appealing or comforting. Parents must create a loving, understanding, encouraging, and cultural environment. Libraries must be built with books and videos with culturally conscious content. Media should be controlled by the parents. Keep the home holistic and free of negativity.

Parents who have the means should consider opening their homes to children in need of adoption. A large number of Afrikan children need homes. It is the community's responsibility to care for these children. What will become of these children? How will their non-parental situation affect the community as a whole? Today many Caucasian families are adopting children born on the Afrikan continent. Diasporic Afrikans with extra income who visit the continent can keep in contact with Afrikans they may have met while visiting. It costs so little to help parents send their children to school or provide meals for a child. Children do not always need to leave the continent for a brighter future. The children are valuable to their society. Poverty stricken communities in Afrika need support which will enable them to help themselves. Removing the children from the Afrikan family is a loss and the community does not always gain. Many diasporic Afrikans have ties with Afrikan communities on the continent. These people can be used as resources to help identify communities in need. I belong to a sister circle. As a group we pay for a child's entire school year in Ghana. I encourage all to see the wholeness of what it means to be Afrikan. It is time to create a global Afrikan community. The great ancestor John Henrik said, "Pan-Afrikanism or Perish". We all have the ability to be Pan-Afrikan holistic parents whether we have biological children or not. All children are the community's children.

Pan-Afrikanism is key to the global Afrikan family's survival. The Afrikan community must be self–reliant. When sending children off to learn architecture, engineering, agriculture, and business, these skills are not solely for the benefit of corporate America. We must build our homeland, Afrika. Afrika has experienced a brain drain. The educated Continental Afrikans leave their homes and bring their knowledge to places such as Europe and the United States. Many Afrikan countries are rebuilding. If Afrikans of the Diaspora are not choosing to invest in Afrika, other non-Afrikan nations will. Now is the time to invest in the Afrikan community. Now is the time to invest in the Afrikan child!

Bibliography

Introduction

1. Noll, Joyce, Elaine. Company of Prophets: African American Psychics, Healers, and Visionaries. St Paul: Llewellyn Publications, 1991.Pg 29

Chapter 1

1. Meads, Karyne and William B. Meads. Sounds That Nurture the Unborn Child. 1 July 2006.<http://www.setiadd.org/articles_bin/art_sounds.htm l>
2. Doumbia, Naomi and Adama Doumbia. The Way of the Elders: West African Spirituality & Tradition. Saint Paul: Llewellyn Publications, 2004.
3. Huttunen, M and P Niskanen. "Penatal Loss of father And Psychiatric Disorders., Arch of Gen Psychiat 35 (1978): 429-31.
4. Fox, Maggie, Reuters. Unborn babies soaked in chemicals, survey finds. 14 July 2005. 1 July 2006.http://www.enn.com/today.html?id=8239
5. Peters, Diane. "Heal Your Home." Black Woman And Child. Spring 2006: 12-13.
6. McDougall, John. Nutrition For Pregnancy. 1 July 2006.< http://www.drmcdougall.com/newsletter/march_april97.ht ml>
7. Odent. Michael. The Rise of Preconceptual Counseling Vs The Decline of Medicalized Care in Pregnancy. 23 Feb. 2002. 1 July 2006. < http://birthpsychology.com/primalhealth/primal10.html>
8. Some, Sobonfu E. Welcoming Spirit Home: Ancient African Teachings to Celebrate Children and Community. Novato, 1999.
9. Goldsmith, July. "Traditional Childbirth." Mothering. Spring 1989.

160

10. Mohammed, Faduma. "Childbirth, Culture, & Choice." Black Woman And Child. Winter 2006: 12+.

Chapter 2

1. Utsey, Monica, Z. "Reclaiming Midwives: Pillars of the Black Community Natural Childbirth Has a Long History in the Black Community".Capital Community. 2005. 12 Dec 2006.<http://www.capitalcommunitynews.com/publicatio ns/eotr/2005-dec/html/ReclaimingMidwives.cfm>.
2. Hogan, Onnie. Lee. Motherwit. New York: Dutton, 1989.
3. Fiscella, K. "Does prenatal care improve birth outcomes: a critical review." Obstetrics and Gynecology. 85 (1995) 68-479.
4. Odent, Michel. The Caesarean. London: Free Association Books, 2004.
5. Blais, Regis. "Are home births safe?" CMAJ. 166(3) (2002). 335-336.

Chapter 3

1. Giraldo, Roberto. "Everyone Reacts Positive on the ELISA Tests for HIV." Continuum (London). Winter 1998: 8-10.
2. Giraldo, Roberto, et al. " Is It Rational To Treat Or Prevent AIDS With Toxic Antiretroviral Drugs In Pregnant Women, Infants, Children And Anybody Else? The Answer is Negative". Continuum (London). Summer 1999: 38-52.
3. Maggiore, Christine. What if everything you thought you knew about AIDS was wrong? The American Foundation for AIDS Alternatives, 1999.
4. GlaxoSmithKline. Prescription Information. 31 Dec. 2006. <http://us.gsk.com/products/assets/us_retrovir_injection.p df>.
5. Naumburg, Estelle, et al. "Prenatal ultrasound examinations and risk of childhood leukaemia: case-control study." BMJ. 320(7230) (2000):282-283.

6. Matthews, Robert. "Ultrasound Scans Linked to Brain Damage in Babies." Epidemiology 12:618 (2001):169-81.
7. Odent, Michel. The Caesarean. London: Free Association Books, 2004.
8. Goer, Henci. The thinking Woman's Guide to a Better Birth. New York: Perigee, 1999.
9. Belizán, Jose, M. and Guillermo Carroli. "Routine episiotomy should be abandoned." BMJ 317(7169) (1998): 1389.
10. Johanson, Richard and Mary Newburn. "Promoting normality in childbirth." BMJ 323 (7322) (2001) :1142-1143.

11. Xu, B , Pekkanen, J and MR Jarvelin. "Obstetric complications and asthma in childhood." J Asthma . 37 (7) (2000) : 589-94
12. Odent, Michael. The Long Term Consequences of How We Are Born. Primal Health Research Newsletter. 7.1 1999.

Chapter 4

1. Some, Sobonfu E. Welcoming Spirit Home: Ancient African Teachings to Celebrate Children and Community. Novato: 1999.
2. Guthrie, Patricia. "Many Cultures Revere Placenta, by product of Childbirth". Cox News Service. 7 July 1999. 31 Dec. 2006. <http://www.tidesoflife.com/placenta.htm>.
3. Mohammed, Faduma. "Childbirth, Culture, & Choice." Black Woman And Child. Winter 2006: 12+.
4. Nyinah, Stella. "Cultural practices in Ghana." World Health. Mar/Apr1997: 220-3.
5. Wilson, Amos, N. Awakening the Natural Genius of Black Children. New York: Afrikan World InfoSystems, 2003.
6. Patel, Hawa. "The Problem Routine Circumcision." Canadian Medial Association Journal 95 (1966): 576-581.
7. Omara, Peggy. Natural Family Living. New York: Pocket Books, 2000.

8. Hand, Eugene. "Circumcision and venereal disease." Archives of Dermatology and Syphilology 60 (1949): 345-6)

9. "Circumcision for the correction of sexual crimes among the Negro race." Maryland Medical Journal 30 (1894) : 345-6.

10. Davis- Floyd, Robbie, and Dumit, Joseph, eds. Cyborg Babies: From Techno-Sex to Techno-Tots. Oxford: Routledge, 1998.

11. Osburne, Nicole. "Formula Facts." Black Woman And Child. Fall 2006:6+.

12. Yaron, Ruth. Super Baby Food. Pecksville: F.J. Roberts Publishing Company, 1998.

13. Omara, Peggy. " a quite place: a tale of two diapers" Mothering. Sept/Oct 2006; 10.

14. Toby, Lewis. "Somali Cultural Profile." Aug 1996 1 Jul 7 2006 <http://www.ethnomed.org/cultures/somali/somali_cp.htm l>

15. Wax, Emily. "African mothers see baby strollers as abhorrent fad tradition of carrying children upheld; 'they can't sit like lumps'." San Francisco Chronicle. 20 May 2004 4 July 2006 < http://www.sfgate.com/cgi-bin/article.cgi?f=/c/a/2004/05/20/MNG6Q6O4LI1.DTL>

16. Fu – Kiau , Bunseki and A. M Lukondo – Wamba . Kindezi: The Kongo Art of Babysitting. Baltimore: Imprint Editions, 1988 .

Chapter 5

1. Omara, Peggy. Natural Family Living. New York: Pocket Books, 2000.

2. Miller, Neil. Z. Vaccines: Are They Really Safe & Effective. Sante Fe: New Atlantean Press, 2004.

3. Cave, Stephanie M and Debra Mitchell. What Your doctor May Not Tell You About Childrens Vaccinations. New York: Time Warner, 2001.

4. Bahar, H. et al. "Development of multiple sclerosis after vaccination against hepatitis B: a study based on human

leucocyte antigen haplotypes". Tissue Antigens. 68(3) (2006): 235-8.

5. Omara, Peggy. "Safety of HPV vaccine questioned" Mothering. Sept/Oct 2006: 26.

6. Ellison, Bryan, J. and Peter H. Deusberg. Why We Will Never Win The War On AIDS. El Cerrioto: Inside Story Communications, 1994.

7. Mendelsohn, Robert, S. How to Raise A Healthy Child In Spite of Your Doctor. New York: Ballantine, 1984.

8. Snow, Loudell, F. "Tradition Health Beliefs and Practices Among Lower Class Black Americans, In Cross Cultural Medicine." The Western Journal of Medicine 139 (1983) ; 820-828.

9. Fett, Sharla, M. Working Cures: Healing, Health, and Power on Southern Slave Plantations. London: Chapel Hill, 2002.

10. Abel, Caroline and Kofi Busia. "An exploratory ethnobotanical study of the practice of herbal medicine by the Akan Peoples of Ghana." Alternative Medicine Review. 10(2) (2005): 112-22.

11. Sawandi, Tariq. "Yorubic Medicine: The Art of divine Herbology." 4 July 2006<http://www.blackherbals.com/Yorubic_Medicine.ht m>

12. Doumbia, Naomi and Adama Doumbia. the Way of The Elders: West African Spirituality & Tradition. Saint Paul: Llewellyn Publications, 2004.

13. Tierra, Lesley. A Kid's Herb Book: for children of all ages. Oregon: Robert D. Reed Publishers, 2005.

14. Romm, Aviva Jill. Naturally Healthy Babies and Children: A commonsense guide to herbal remedies, nutrition, and health. Berkeley: Celestial Arts, 2003.

15. Universtity of Nebraska Medical Center, "Nursing Facts.", 24 Aug 2006 <http://www.unmc.edu/nursing/careers/nurse_facts.htm>

16. Kurokawa, Y, et al. "Long-term in Vivo Carcinogenicity Tests of Potassium Bromate, Sodium Hypochiorite, and Sodium Chlorite Conducted in Japan." Environmental Health Perspectives 69 (1986) : 221-35.

17. Vorhees, CV. "Developmental toxicity and psychotoxicity of FD and C red dye No. 40 (allura red AC) in rats." Toxicology. 28(3) (1983) : 207-17.
18. Peters, Diane. "Eating organic: for the health of your family." Black Woman And Child. Spring 2006: 9-10.

Chapter 6

1. Peters, Diane. "Heal Your Home." Black Woman And Child. Spring 2006: 11-13.
2. Swain, Rachel. "baby and the bath water." Mothering. Mar/Apr 2006: 49-55.
3. Doumbia, Naomi and Adama Doumbia. the Way of The Elders: West African Spirituality & Tradition. Saint Paul: Llewellyn Publications, 2004.
4. King, Cherie. Her Special Hare: A Guide To Understanding and Caring For Your Biracial of African – American daughter's HIGHLY Texturized Hair. Detroit: Crowning Glory Natural Hair Publications, 2006.
5. Kulvinskas, Viktoras. Survival Into The 21st Century. Connecticut: Omangod Press, 1975.

Chapter 7

1. Wilson, Amos, N. Awakening the Natural Genius of Black Children. New York: Afrikan World InfoSystems, 2003.
2. Dove, Nah . Afrikan Mothers: Bearers of Culture, Makers of Social Change. New York: State University of New York, 1998.
3. Kunjufu, Jawanza. Countering the Conspiracy to destroy Black boys Series. Chicago: African American Images, 2005.
4. McGrandle, P.W. "great green schools" Mothering. May/June 2006: 63-65.
5. Omara, Peggy. Natural Family Living. New York: Pocket Books, 2000.

Index

Abosom, 6, 7, 9, 99
Activated charcoal, 109
Africa, 76
Afrika, 28, 60, 64, 72, 86, 91, 96, 117, 122, 126, 139, 157, 158, 159
AIDS, 37, 38, 39, 88
Air, 152
Alfalfa, 19, 116
All In Ones, 70, 71
Allopathic, 94
Altar, 20
Aluminum, 126
Amos Wilson, 144, 149
Anise, 99
Antibiotics, 31, 95
Ants, 126
Apple, 118
Appliances, 123
Aspartame, 113
Assata Shakur, 122
Auset, 19, 22, 28
Autoimmune disorders, 87
AZT, 39
B-12, 18, 115, 116, 120
Baby, 66, 75, 76, 84
Baby wearing, 75
Baby-sit, 84
Basil, 99
Beans, 18
BHA, 112
BHT, 112
Biomass, 139
Birth, 28, 32, 33, 35, 36, 42, 43, 46, 47, 48, 52
Birth Plan, 32
Blackstrap molasses, 19
Blessing Way, 21, 22
Blood Pressure, 107, 108
Bovine Growth Hormone, 120
Breast, 66, 67
Breast milk, 66, 67
Breastfeeding, 63, 64, 66
Buganda, 21
Burkina Faso, 58
Burns, 99

Burritos, 121
Caesarean, 43, 47
Calcium, 19
Calendula, 99
Canada, 146
Capsule, 99
Catnip, 99
Cayenne, 99, 110
CDC, 38, 89, 92
Celery, 112, 118
Cervidil, 41
Chamomile, 99
Chickenpox, 90
Childbirth, 37
Cinnamon, 100, 122
Circumcision, 60, 61, 62
Cloth Diapering, 69
Clove, 100
Cockroaches, 125
Colds, 101
Colic, 100
Cough, 100
CPR, 107
Crystals, 15
Culture, 145, 153
Cytotec, 41
Dagara, 20, 21
Dairy, 17, 120, 121
Daycare, 76, 84, 86
Daylight, 148
DDT, 13, 91
Decoctions, 103
Demoral, 41
Diaper Covers, 71
Diapers, 70, 71
Diaspora, 60, 99, 143, 144, 159
Diet, 16, 148
Diodes, 15, 124
Diphtheria, 89
Disease, 38, 90
Doula, 34
DTaP, 92
DTP, 92
Earaches, 100
Earth, 35, 36, 148
Echinacea, 100, 110

Economics, 153
Education, 140, 142, 144
Egypt, 15
Electricity, 138
Electromagnetic Radiation, 14
Electronic Fetal Monitoring, 42
Elegba, 99, 100, 101
ELFs, 15
Emergencies, 108, 109
EMFs, 15, 124
Environmental Working Group, 13, 126
Episiotomy, 42
Essential Fatty Acids, 115
Essential oils, 126, 129
Eyes, 106
Falafels, 121
Fatherhood, 154
FDA, 38, 41, 46
Fentanyl, 41
Fetal monitoring, 41
Fever, 106
Fire, 9, 109
Flaxseed Oil, 115
Fleas, 125
Flu, 99, 101
Fluoride, 126
Food Coloring, 113
Formaldehyde, 129
Formula, 64
Frankincense, 122
Furniture Polish, 125
Galactagogues, 66
Garlic, 100
Geb, 11
Genetically Modified Foods, 114
George Washington Carver, 9
Ghana, 8, 58, 96, 122, 158
Ginger, 100, 110
Goldenseal, 110
Green leafy vegetables, 18
Guanidine Hydroxide, 128
Haemophilus Influenzae Type B, 90
Hair, 128, 129, 131
Hair Care, 128
Hair relaxers, 128
Harriet Tubman, 122
Hepatitis B, 32, 92

Herbalism, 96, 153
Herbs, 26, 66, 96
Heru, 20, 29
Het Heru, 29, 98
High Fructose Corn Syrup, 113
HIV, 37, 38, 39, 88
Homeschool, 149
Homeschooling, 144, 148, 149, 151
Hospital, 28, 31, 45
HPV, 92
Hummus, 121
Induction, 40
Infant, 64, 142
Ipecac, 109, 110
Irish moss, 19, 119
Iron, 19, 120
IV, 31, 33, 41
John Coltrane, 20, 122, 142
Juicing, 117, 118
Kary Mullis, 38
Kenya, 143
Khemit, 15
Kikuyu, 143
Kirikou and the Sorceress, 133
Knitting, 155
Kwame Nkrumah, 122
Labor, 49, 50
Libation, 58
Licorice, 100
Loa, 6, 9, 99
Lye, 128
Maat, 8, 70, 119
Malachite, 16
Mali, 12, 55, 64, 127
Measles, 89
Meningitis, 90
Mercury, 13
Meshkenet, 29
Mice, 125, 126
Midwife, 25, 26, 29, 35
Midwifery, 25, 26, 28, 48
Milk, 17, 66
MMR, 89
Moonstone, 15, 16
Motherhood, 155
Mucus, 17, 106
Mullein, 100
Mumps, 89
Mut, 7, 19, 149, 150

Nana Esi Ketewaa., 29
Narcotics, 41
Nature, 153
Nausea, 100
Neter, 6, 99
Netert, 19
Nettle, 66
Newborn, 32
Nigeria, 58
Nina Simone, 20
Nu, 22
Nubane, 41
Nutritional Yeast, 115
Nuts, 19, 116
Nyama, 12
Obstetrician and Gynecologist, 25, 27
Ogun, 100
Oils, 104
Omega 3, 19, 115
Omega 6, 19
Omega 9, 19
Onions, 105
Onnie Lee Hogan, 26, 29
Organic, 67, 118, 148
Orisha, 99
Orunmilla, 100, 101
Oshun, 29, 98, 99, 100, 101
Otoscope, 107
Oya, 7, 99, 100, 101
Pain, 40
Pan-Afrikanism, 158, 159
Parasites, 100
Pediatrician, 94
Peppermint, 101, 110
Pertussis, 91
Pest Control, 124
Pesticides, 13, 114, 148
PFOA, 13
Phthalates, 127
Pitocin, 40, 46
PKU, 32, 94
Placenta, 58
Plantain, 101, 110
Plants, 123
Pneumonia, 39
Poison Prevention, 109
Polio, 91
Polyvinyl Chloride, 121

Postpartum, 58
Potassium Bromate, 112
Prefolds, 70
Pregnancy, 16
Protein, 19
Puerto Rico, 8, 36
Pulse, 107, 108
PVC, 121, 127
Quaternium-15, 129
Queen Nzinga, 122
Quinoa, 117
Ra, 3, 11, 28, 53, 55, 64
Radio, 133
Raw Food, 111
Red 40, 113
Red Raspberry, 66
Respiration Rate, 107, 108
Retrovirals, 39
Rubella, 89
Safflower oil, 19
Sage, 101
Schooling, 149, 150
Schools, 144, 147, 148
Seeds, 116
Senegal, 12, 98, 127
Sewing, 155
Sexuality, 154, 155
Shampoos, 126
Shango, 99
Shu, 11
Slippery Elm, 101, 115
Smoothies, 119
Sodium Hydroxide, 128
Sodium Nitrate, 113
Solar energy, 137
Somalia, 21, 59, 72
Soups, 50, 121
Spice, 100, 101
Spinach, 114, 118
Sprouts, 116, 117
Stadol, 41
Standard American Diet, 119
STDs, 61
Stephen Bantu Biko, 122
Sugar, 121
Sun Ra, 20, 142
Sunlight, 18
Sustainable Living, 122
Syrups, 104

Tea, 99, 100, 101, 103, 105, 111
Tea tree oil, 111
Teflon, 13
Tefnut, 11
Television, 133, 135
Tetanus, 88
Thyme, 101
Toddler, 142
Toys, 127
Twi, 149, 154
Ugandan, 60, 143
Ukanite, 16
Unassisted, 25, 26
United Kingdom, 8, 144, 146
United States, 8, 13, 28, 38, 43, 44, 60, 87, 89, 91, 143, 145, 146, 159
Vaccinations, 87, 88, 93
Vaccine, 88
Valerian, 111
Vegan, 16, 17, 119, 121
Violence, 154
Vital sign, 107

Vitamin A, 18
Vitamin B, 18
Vitamin B 12, 18
Vitamin B 6, 18
Vitamin B 9, 18
Vitamin C, 18
Vitamin D, 18
Vitamin E, 18
Vitamin K, 19, 33
Vodka, 104
Wailers, 20
Water, 8, 12, 15, 21, 28, 56, 121
West Africa, 58
Wheat Germ, 115
Wheatgrass, 116
Whole grain, 18, 67
Womb, 11
Wood, 127
Wounds, 101
Yellow dock, 17
Yemaya, 20, 22, 28, 53, 99, 100, 101
Yoruba, 20, 99, 149, 154

169

For more Books, Publishing & Printing Information

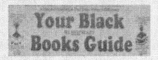 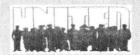

"The KHA WAY – Quality & Quickly!"

Go to:
www.khabooks.com e-mail publish@khabooks.com

WRITE OR CALL

 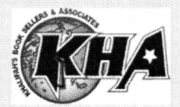

KHA ONLINE BOOKSELLERS
www.khalifahandassociates
Charlotte, North Carolina 28213

KHABOOKS
P. O. Box 9
Drewryville, Virginia 23844

(704) 509-2226   or (704) 277-1462